I0755839

Smart, Beautiful and Important

Smart, Beautiful and Important

Teaching art to AIDS-affected orphans in Africa's largest slum

By Charles DeSantis

Foreword by
Margaret Halpin

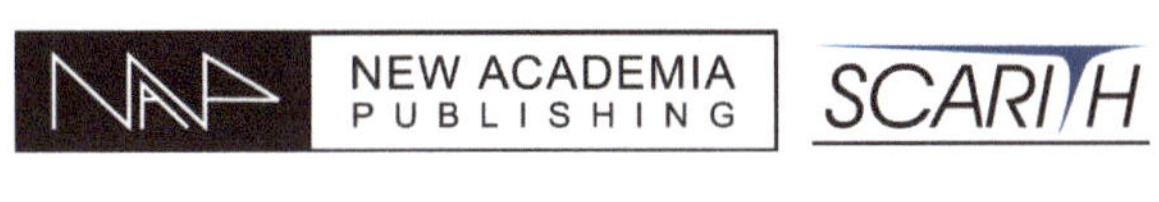

Washington, DC

New Academia Publishing, 2010

Printed in the United States of America

Library of Congress Control Number: 2010931475
ISBN 978-0-9828061-1-1 hardcover (alk. paper)

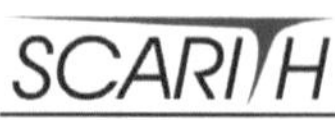

SCARITH is an imprint of New Academia Publishing

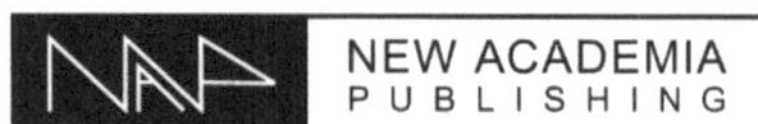

P.O. Box 27420, Washington, DC, 30028-7420
info@newacademia.com - www.newacademia.com

100% of all proceeds from the sale of this book wil benefit
St. Aloysius Gonzaga High School in Nairobi.

This book is for my mother Mary DeSantis who loves me
no matter what, believes in my unlimited potential and
who has taught me to live a life of gratitude.

For my sister Anna Badger and brother Michael DeSantis
whom I love very much.

For my father Anthony R. DeSantis, Jr. who is no longer
here on earth, but whose support and love I still feel every day.

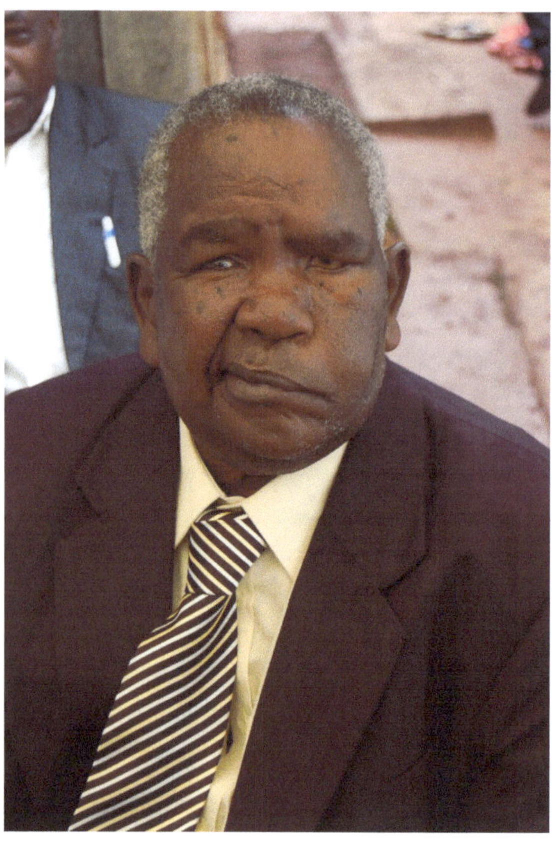

In remembrance of Samuel Ndirangu Waweru who died on July 25, 2010, the same day I completed this book. The father of my dearest friend, Anne Wangari, Samuel became my Kenyan father (Awa) and graciously welcomed me into his family. I saw Samuel as a wonderful representative of the Kenyan people and their loving spirit; may this book honor his memory and those that hold it dear. And, although it may go without saying, may this book also serve as a tribute to the Smart, Beautiful and Important students of St. Aloysius Gonzaga Secondary School in Nairobi.

FOREWORD

What happens when you bring a contemporary U.S.-style visual arts program to a high school for AIDS orphans in the heart of one of Africa's largest slums?

Art Education has had many justifications over the course of its history in the United States. According to Elliott Eisner, those justifications have included: avocational, physiological, therapeutic; a tool for the development of creative thinking or a hand maiden to concept formation in academic subject areas. Art education as an inclusion in the K-12 curriculum was justified as utilitarian as early as 1749 by Benjamin Franklin, or a vehicle for communication, at times society centered, child centered, or subject centered.

This is a success story about art as social justice in Kibera, Nairobi, Kenya. Kibera is a harsh, impoverished environment. It struggles, albeit optimistically, for democracy, equity, equality, and economic development amidst tribal conflicts and difficulties to meet basic human needs for water, food and shelter.

In 2007, Charles and I were invited to participate in a trip sponsored by Georgetown University to be immersed in the many social justice challenges facing the people in and around Nairobi, Kenya, mostly through the many programs supported by faith-based initiatives. Little did I know that a passion for art and a long time curiosity about Africa would come together in an initiative to teach art to AIDS orphans in the massive slum of Kibera.

Charles DeSantis and I met on that 2007 trip to Kenya. Early on we discovered we had a mutual interest in the arts, he as a painter and teacher and I as an art educator, but our careers had taken us into administration, he as Associate Vice President and Chief Benefits Officer and me as an Associate Dean for Finance and Administration in the School of Foreign Service, both at Georgetown University. I was aware of Charles as a dynamic and endearing change agent on campus, a man who gets things done.

Kibera is a slum of about one million people who live in structures made mostly of mud covered with tin roofs with little or no running water or electricity. The raw sewage accumulates in the paths between structures. St. Aloysius Gonzaga High School for AIDS-affected children was located down one of these sewage strewn paths, an oasis of safety and education, in an extremely difficult community. On the day we first visited St. Al's we walked single file down a wet, muddy, malodorous path. Charles walked behind me. I made an attempt to try to help a colleague who was carrying a heavy book while walking with a cane. I was the one who slipped and fell in the muck. Charles stopped me as I was about to wipe the muck from my pants with bare hands. He saved me from exposing myself further to an environment that would be hostile for a non-native like me. We went on to tour the school. In our discussions independently and almost simultaneously we inquired if there was an art program. We learned that no, there was not. Would they like an arts program? Well, yes of course, but there was not enough time in the day to include this in the curriculum. Charles suggested that maybe we could do something about that and the idea was born to deliver a program between academic sessions. We spent the next year meeting weekly to discuss and plan how to deliver an intensive art immersion program at St. Al's. We pondered the

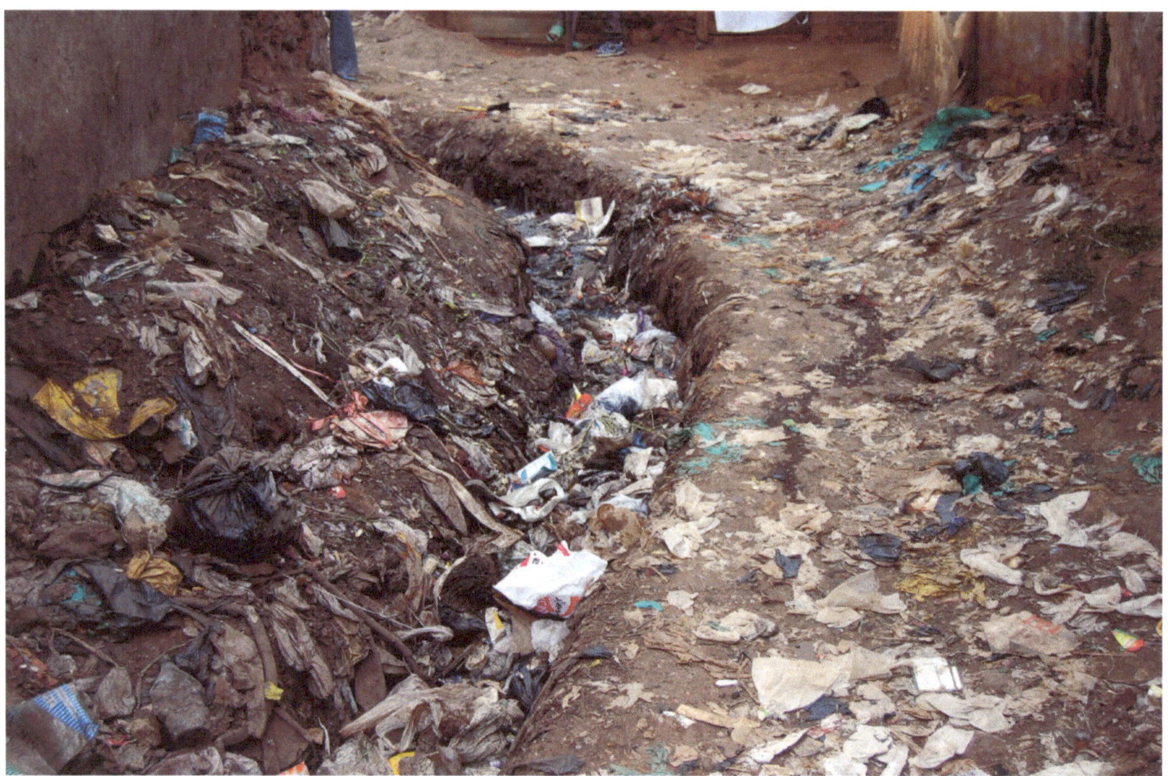

Sewage strewn pathway to St. Al's School in Kibera.

question: If you only have two weeks–and this may be the only art program these students will ever have–what do you cover? We assembled a curriculum to cover basic art history and appreciation topics as well as to allow students to experience the creative process in a variety of media such as drawing, painting and photography.

Charles had the forethought to start a blog as we embarked on our first trip. At the end of each day we eagerly talked about curriculum, students, and general observations. He would passionately chronicle the events and observations and read it to me before he hit the enter button. The blog tells the tale in a mix of travelogue sprinkled with keen and immediate descriptions of the social and economic conditions. It also shares the joys and frustrations of teaching art in a slum intermixed with side adventures with elephants, Kenyan scouts, food, and new friends.

Since embarking on this adventure, I have often wondered why it has all worked so well. Certainly a good part of the success is because Charles is "amazing." People

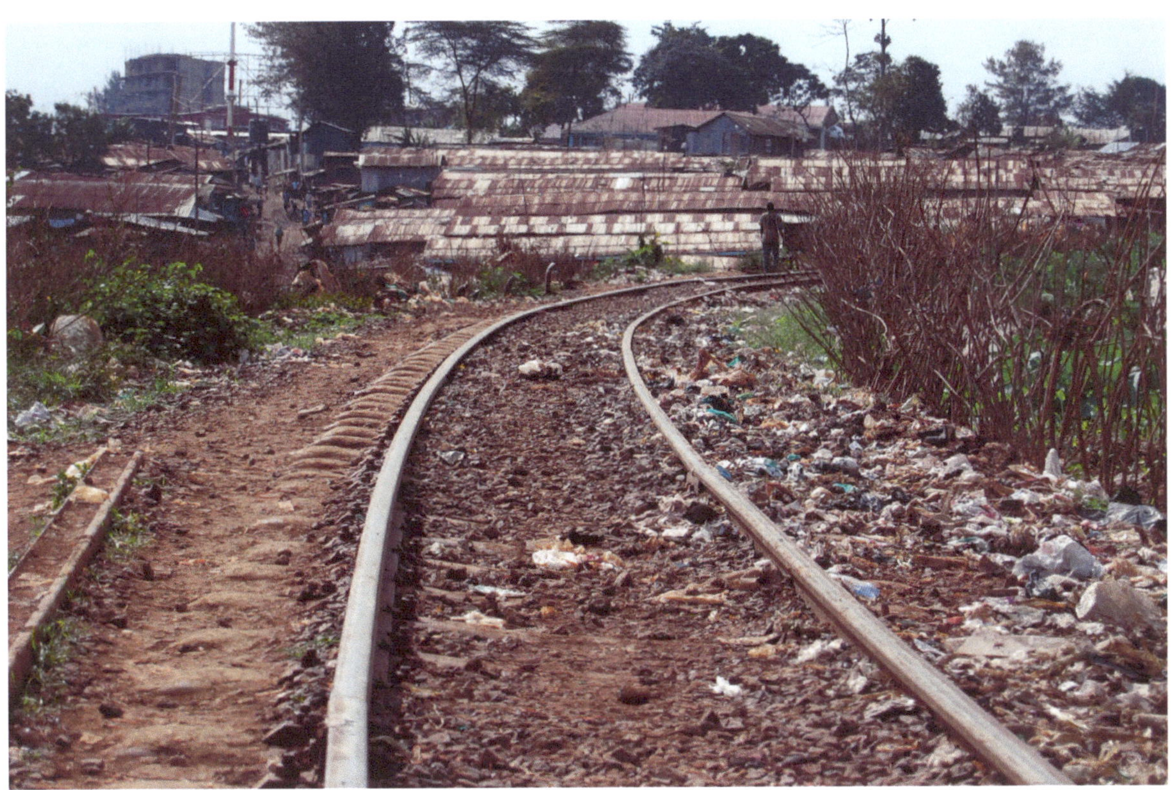

Outskirts of the Kibera slum in Nairobi, Kenya.

have asked me: *Why are you doing this project in Africa? Why not do something here in the United States?* My response is that, much to my amazement, all the pieces fell into place for this initiative. In that sense, I believe there are forces at work that we are just enabling to happen. We have not forced our ideas. We were invited, we were moved by personal passion, and we were willing to make the effort without financial compensation.

Charles has captured our experience as it occurred with all its raw excitement and emotion. Sometimes naive and sometimes deeply insightful it reveals the revelations, joys, puzzlements and wonder experienced on a daily basis. I believe there is so much more to explore and that this initiative will endure. To use Charles's favorite descriptor, this is an "amazing" journey about social justice and art in Kibera. It is only the beginning.

Margaret Halpin

INTRODUCTION

When I first received an invitation to take part in an immersion experience in Africa I never thought it would result in the creation of an art program for AIDS orphans in the Kibera Slum of Nairobi. Even more than chronicling the journey of creating and delivering an art program, this story is about the incredible power of reciprocity and engagement.

Who knew that my life-long love of art and my art practice and educational background would end up serving a set of the poorest young people in Kenya's largest slum? If I never believed that providence existed before, I do now. As I write this, I find myself as shocked (and delighted!) by the events that have transpired as I was when I was first asked to participate. I want to share the story that got me to this place, this moment.

In my senior year of high school, while composing a senior thesis on apartheid, my mind suddenly, and for the first time, shifted its perspective from local to global. It dawned on me that there are things happening in the world of which I am totally unaware. As I wrote this paper and really began to comprehend this issue of apartheid, a seed of hope was planted that one day I would do relief work that would result in making a difference in what I saw as a challenging, flawed and horrible existence for so many. I thought that this would be work I would pursue in my retirement. My naïve, 18-year old self did not in any way know what it would look like to do relief work in Africa. We've all seen Sally Struthers urging us to give money to the malnourished children in Africa, but I really had no idea what that meant. I went on to college, started my life and never put more thought into it.

Fast forward nearly 20 years to 2006: Now a senior administrator at Georgetown University, I was asked by Phil Boroughs, SJ and Kathleen Maas Weigert, Ph.D. to take part in a Kenya Immersion Program sponsored by their respective divisions within, and with the support of, the University. I had to stop and ask myself "how did they know that I would like to work in Africa?" It was unbelievable. I had to consider that my recent appointment at Georgetown may have been in even greater alignment with my future goals than I could imagine. I excitedly accepted their invitation and started to gear up for a trip to Kenya that would change my life forever.

Arriving in Nairobi in June of 2007 for a two-week sojourn through the good and bad of Kenya really changed my lens. I met some of the most beautiful, loving and smart people that I could have imagined. They were the people we met in the slums. The first day after our arrival we visited St. Joseph the Worker Parish in the Kengami slum. I mention this specifically because it was the first defining moment relating to why I had been asked to come on this trip. As we were returning to the

Toddler in Kengami.

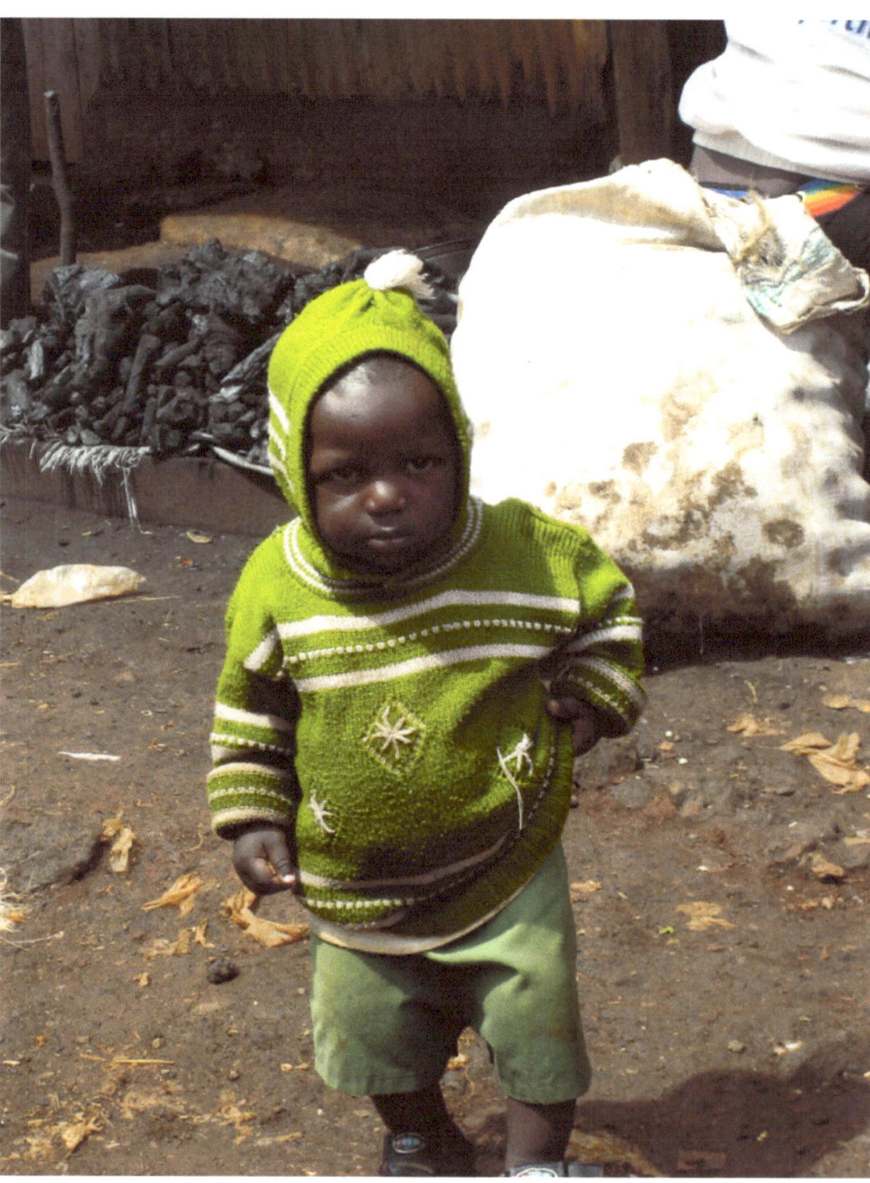

vans after walking through the parish and its surrounding community in Kengami, a few of us veered off to the left when everyone else was walking to the right. I was distracted by a beautiful toddler in a green sweater who looked at me with a beautiful, hopeful, tired and worn out all-in-one expression. At that moment I realized, if there is only one reason for me to be on this trip to Kenya, it would be to somehow help these beautiful children. I was overwhelmed by the emotion I felt as I looked at this child. Even at this point, I still didn't really comprehend what this all meant to me. Against the guidance we had been given, I pulled out my camera and took pictures of this beautiful toddler, and then I went and rejoined the group.

Throughout that trip we experienced many harsh realities. We saw the place where homeless young boys who had been sniffing glue to alleviate their hunger and calm their minds were given refuge; we saw anguished refugees without identity, community or sense of belonging; the Nyumbani orphanage (the first orphanage for children with AIDS); and we saw the Kibera Slum.

You can imagine that this was an overwhelming experience. Yet the recurring theme was one of hope–there were so many individuals engaged in making a difference. When we first entered Kibera, I realized that I had never seen anything like this. The abject poverty, squalor, children walking barefoot through raw sewage, and smells overwhelmed me. Awkwardly, what struck me most was the hope and beauty that I saw in these Kenyans. As we moved through this community, the thought that these people were displays on a tour made me nauseous; as we moved through Kibera, I had to change that immediately for myself. I started to engage each person by saying *hello* and *how are you.* The response was lovely. In a sing song voice, you would hear them say *Hello, how are you, I am fine*. Now I felt better. We were in their territory and I felt we should engage and let them know that we were there to understand their issues. That was not accomplished in reality, only in my mind as I continued to engage each and every person we met. By the time we arrived at the St. Aloysius of Gonzaga Secondary School, I was mentally spent.

When I walked into the school with its corrugated roof and dirt floors and saw these young people so intensely engaged in learning and so hungry for it, I was shocked. They wanted to be there. They wanted their education and they knew that education was the gateway to possibility. In reviewing their curriculum, I could not find any indication that they created visual arts. When I inquired about it, I was told that the government sets the curriculum and art is not part of it.

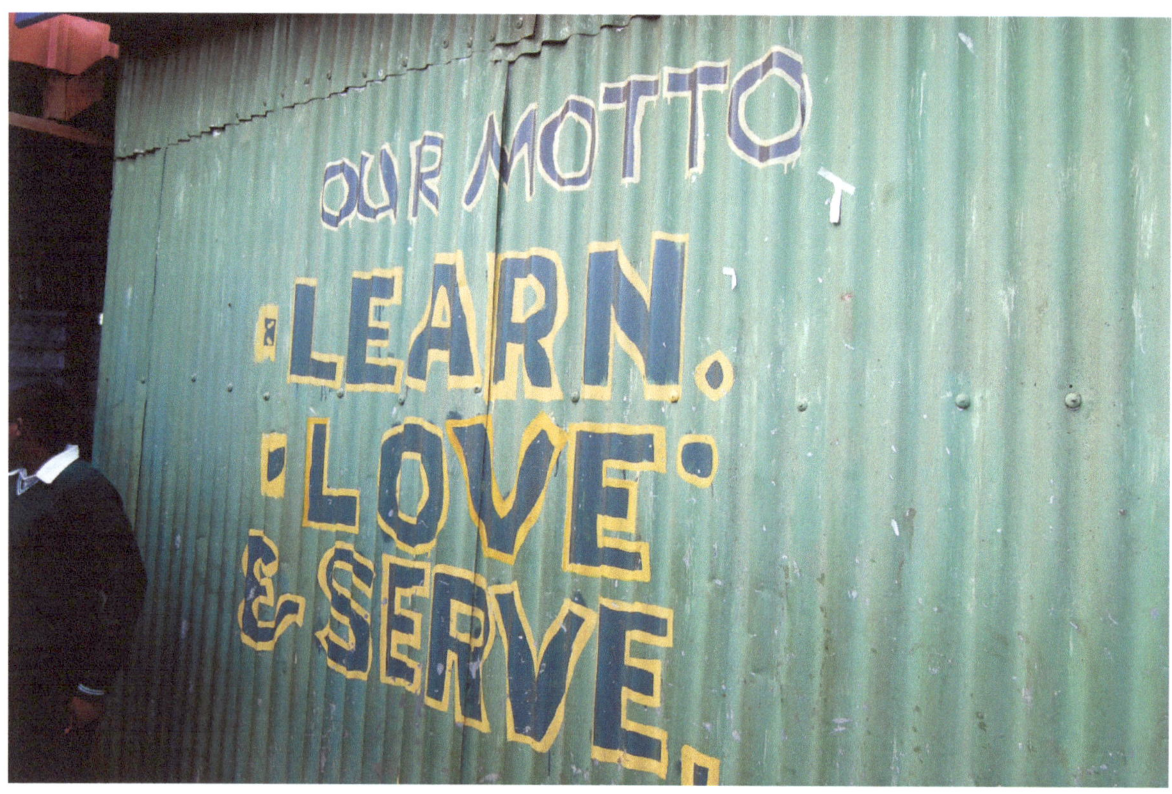

St. Aloysius Gonzaga High School for AIDS-affected children.

I was also told that if I wanted to create a program, they would be open to it. Little did I know that within the same hour that I had that conversation so did Margaret. During our group debrief that evening, Margaret and I discovered that we both had made the same inquiry, both heard the same response and both had art backgrounds. We regarded each other with confusion and excitement as we declared that we believed we could create a meaningful program that we could deliver in a truncated amount of time. We just didn't know how.

After a year of planning and fundraising, we delivered the first Art Immersion program to the smart, beautiful and important students of St. Al's in August 2008 and this is where this story begins. This book was created from the daily blog entries of the three years we delivered this program to date. I wrote, Margaret reviewed and, now, we are delighted to share it with you. There are two things that I hope you will take away from this story: You never know what will make a difference in someone's life; and, one person at a time can absolutely make a difference. Throughout our first trip to Kenya, these were the themes that kept resurfacing as the many people we encountered made a difference in the lives of so many. An important life lesson I learned on that trip was that you never know how you might make a difference in someone life, and what that might look like, until you show up and figure it out. I never imagined that I would be delivering art education to AIDS orphans in the Kibera slum. On that same point, I never thought I would be publishing a book about the program.

As I sit here writing this introduction, Margaret and I just returned from our third year of delivering this art immersion program in Nairobi. What an amazing experience! Never underestimate your ability to make a difference. Because, chances are, you probably already have made a difference in someone's life, one person at a time, and you may not even know it.

With gratitude,

Charles

July 25, 2010

ART IN KIBERA

NAIROBI, KENYA 2008

WEDNESDAY, AUGUST 6, 2008
36 hours until we leave for Nairobi.

Margaret Halpin and I are just 36 hours away from to the start of our journey to teach at St. Al's in the Kibera slum of Nairobi, Kenya. I know it will be an amazing experience and, although it feels like there is so much to do, I trust we will get on that plane at 11 pm on Thursday night fully prepared for the experience.

We'll be teaching art to Forms 1 and 2 (that translates to 9th and 10th graders) who don't have access to any sort of art education. St. Al's serves AIDS orphans in a college preparatory environment right in the middle of the largest slum on the continent of Africa. The Kibera slum, which is about one square mile with no traditional running water or electricity, is home to 1 million people.

These beautiful people are so hopeful and full of life. It is exciting to be able to teach them something that they don't have access to; something that will help them to think and visualize the world differently than they do today. I never imagined that when I went to art school – almost 20 years ago now! - it would lead me to a slum in Nairobi. The old adage is true: anything is possible. You can never predict how your life experiences will impact you, or others.

Both Margaret and I have art backgrounds. She was an NEA Fellow and art teacher for twelve years. I am an artist who studied painting, had a residency at The San Francisco Art Institute and taught art to kindergarteners for two years.

While we're in Nairobi we'll be staying at the Savelberg Retreat Center and will have a driver named Franco. Both the accommodations and the driver have been arranged for by my dear friend, Anne Wangari. It's incredible how things just seem to come together; I am grateful for everyone's support.

As we are able, Margaret and I will try to keep the blog up-to-date. At this point we are unclear as to whether we'll have email access.

Be well and thanks to all of you who've been so supportive of our art adventure in Kenya!

Charles and Margaret

THURSDAY, AUGUST 7, 2008
We leave today.

Just want to let you know that, speaking for myself, I am packed and ready to go. There are only very minor things left to do. To give you a sense of the process, however, I must disclose that I was on the phone with Margaret last night well after 11pm discussing appropriate wardrobe options. That might give you a little insight into our night of prep.

We look forward to sharing wonderful stories with you and hope to be able to keep this blog as up-to-date as possible.

Thanks to you all for the support that you've provided to make this trip a reality.

Be Well,

Charles and Margaret

SATURDAY, AUGUST 9, 2008
It feels like we have returned home.

Margaret and I landed in Nairobi today and were greeted by our new friend (and driver for the next few weeks), Franco Sego. Thanks to Anne Wangari for making the arrangements.

Aside from Margaret's bout of suspected food poisoning on the DC to London leg of our trip, we arrived in one piece. We had an eight-hour layover in Heathrow and, thanks to Margaret's pre-flight research, we were able to relax, sleep and watch the Olympics in the ServiceAir lounge for only a few, well-spent dollars.

This is really happening. I think it really sank in for both of us when we first met Franco. It was really nice to have someone pick us up. I must say that having only two people to maneuver made the process much easier when compared to our inaugural visit to Kenya last year with fourteen of our Georgetown colleagues. I realize that Jan (who organized the Kenya Immersion trip last year) should be granted sainthood for herding us University-types through Kenya.

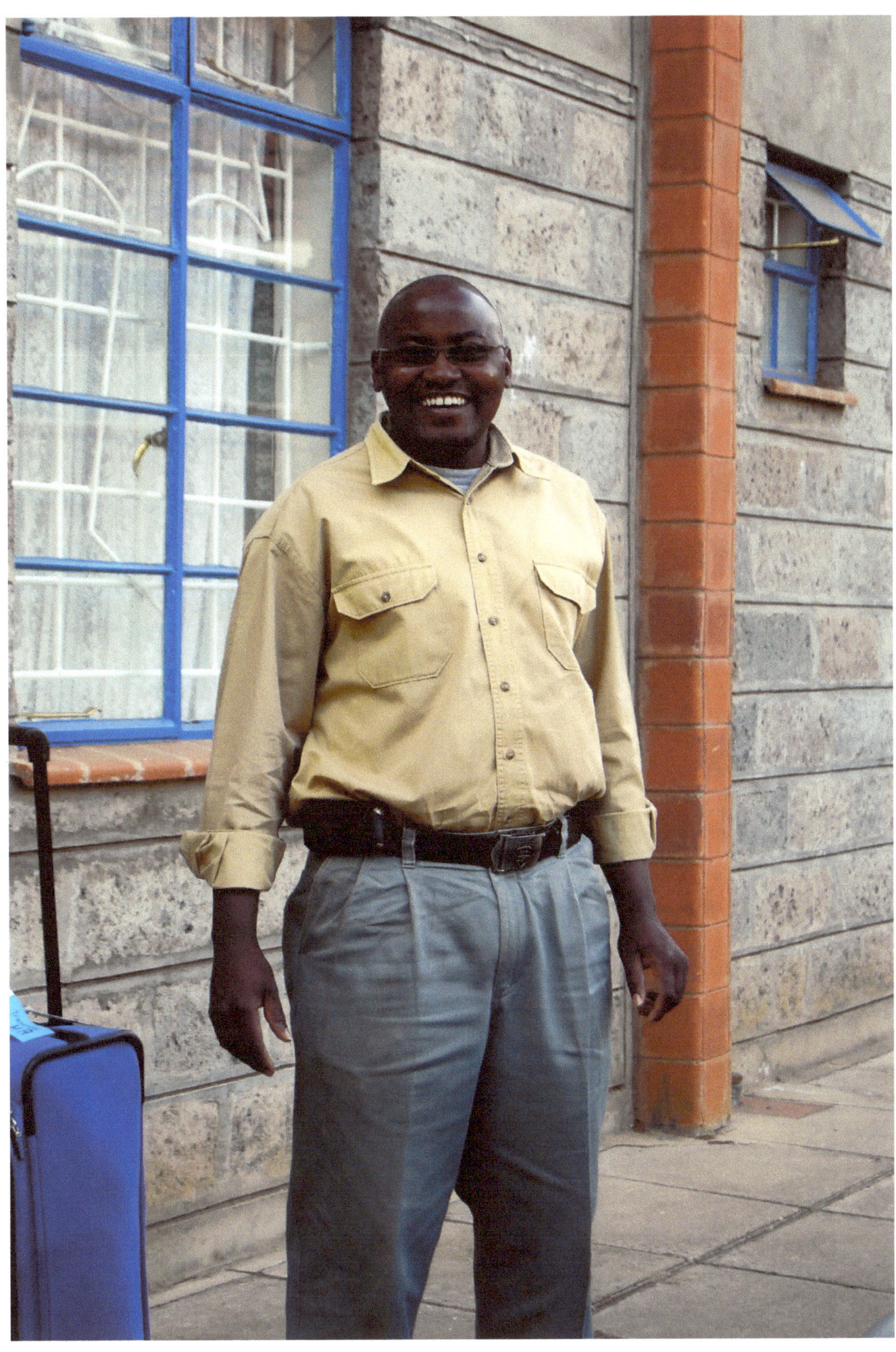

Our driver, tour guide and friend, Franco Sego.

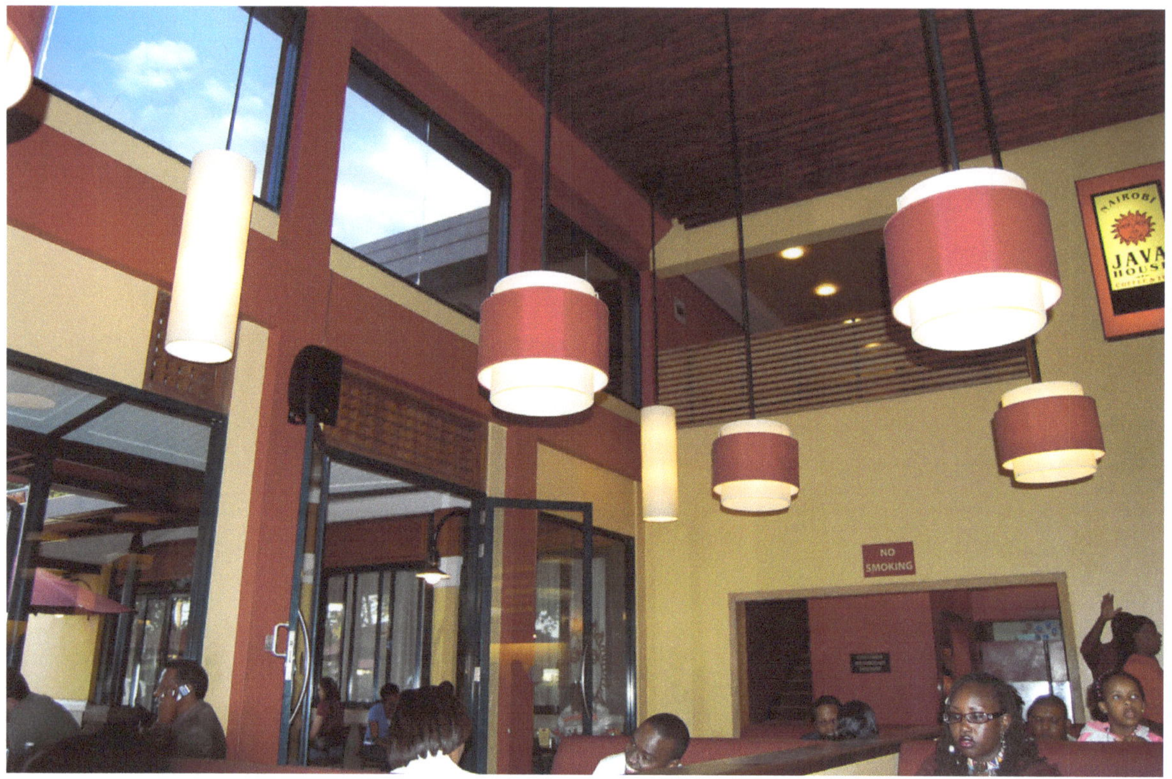

Nairobi Java, our home away from home.

We checked in to warm and welcoming accommodations at the Savelberg Retreat Center - just blocks away from the Loyola House where we will dine with Father Superior of East Africa, Valerian Shirima next Saturday. He is a great man and head of the Jesuits for East Africa.

After we checked in we started our day at, of all places, Nairobi Java. This is, essentially, a diner with great food and amazing coffee and, although it is very Kenyan, has a distinct appeal to the western set. Everyone knows of Nairobi Java as there are many located around the city. You can buy burgers and the like; my favorite are the samosas. Yum.

From there, it was off to Nakumatt. This is the greatest "all things" store, ever. We needed to stock up on water and snacks to assure that we don't starve. Although I think I could use a good week of starvation, we need to make sure Margaret eats every meal!

After shopping we went to Pedro Arrupe (a Jesuit home and retreat center where we had stayed during our 2007 visit) and had tea with Deborah Moijoi.

Deborah is the administrator of Pedro Arrupe; she's a Masai woman who lives in the adjacent community across the river in the Rift Valley region with her family. She always treated us with such warmth and openness. Her booming sing-song voice is unmistakable, "Oh dear Lord! Charles and Margaret, what are you doing here?!" We enjoyed catching up over tea and made plans to see her family next weekend. We also had the privilege of meeting Fr. Jim, head of Pedro Arrupe, another great man I hope we may see at Nyumbani tomorrow.

Next, we went on the overwhelming adventure that is the Kazuri Jewelry Factory tour and shop. Kazuri jewelry is hand-made, hand-painted ceramic jewelry made exclusively by 350 women who work in this Nairobi factory. It's beautifully colorful and expressive stuff. I resisted but Margaret made a great purchase.

From Kazuri we returned to Savelberg for some rest. Now we are headed back to Nairobi Java for a nice dinner.

As I expressed in my conversations with Margaret today, it feels like we have returned home. I never thought I would feel this way about Kenya. Home has always been where my family is. Being a Navy brat, home moves, and for me, home has moved many, many times. Now it's moved to Kenya.

Good news: we have internet via both Nairobi Java and Savelberg so we will be able to update the blog often.

Best wishes and
Be well,

Charles and Margaret

MONDAY, AUGUST 11, 2008
Wow and more wow. That's all we can say.

Sunday started off early with Mass at Nyumbani Orphange. At Nyumbani (which means 'home' in Swahili) children are cared for until a definite assessment of their HIV status can be made. Children who are eventually found not to have the virus are adopted or find other homes. Children who are found to be HIV+ are given the best nutritional, medical (specifically, anti-retroviral therapy) psychological, academic, and spiritual care available. They live at Nyumbani until they become self-reliant. The Kenya 2007 group did not have an opportunity to see the grounds due to intense rains. Seeing it now, I'm amazed at the juxtaposition of such incredible beauty against such a harsh reality. Out of 106 children, 105 are healthy

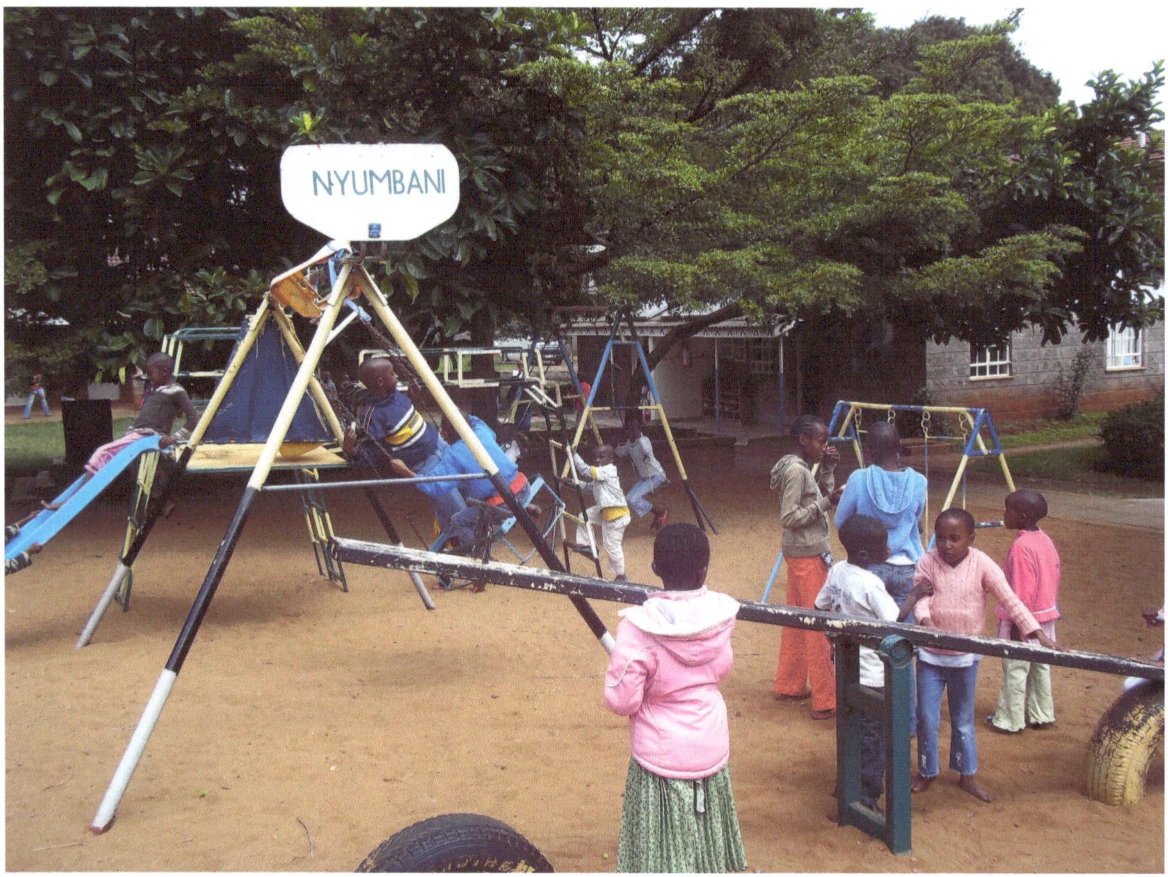

Nyumbani Orphanage serves as home to 106 children who are HIV-positive.

and one is dying. Sammy has 24-hour care and is really sick. Your heart just sinks knowing that a terminal outcome is imminent and that there's nothing you can do to help. Those that are part of Nyumbani have dedicated their lives to the care and love of these HIV+ children. I can only imagine how hard, helpless and wrong it must seem when a child dies. Sr. Mary Owens, the executive director of Nyumbani, was gracious enough to introduce us at Mass. As you might expect, it was a very child-centric service. The kids acted, sang, danced, and at the end of it all, they looked really loved. After Mass we met a woman from Williams College who, after working to adopt a child from Nyumbani for two years, will be returning home to Massachusetts with her new son, Bernard, in a week. She is the first person to adopt an HIV+ child from Kenya. She has been on leave in Kenya for two years and now it is becoming a reality for her. What an amazing story.

Kibera is a little easier for me this time around. At least, this time, I know what to expect. I think for Margaret it is still as hard as the first time. It's really difficult to know that these beautiful people live in such squalor.

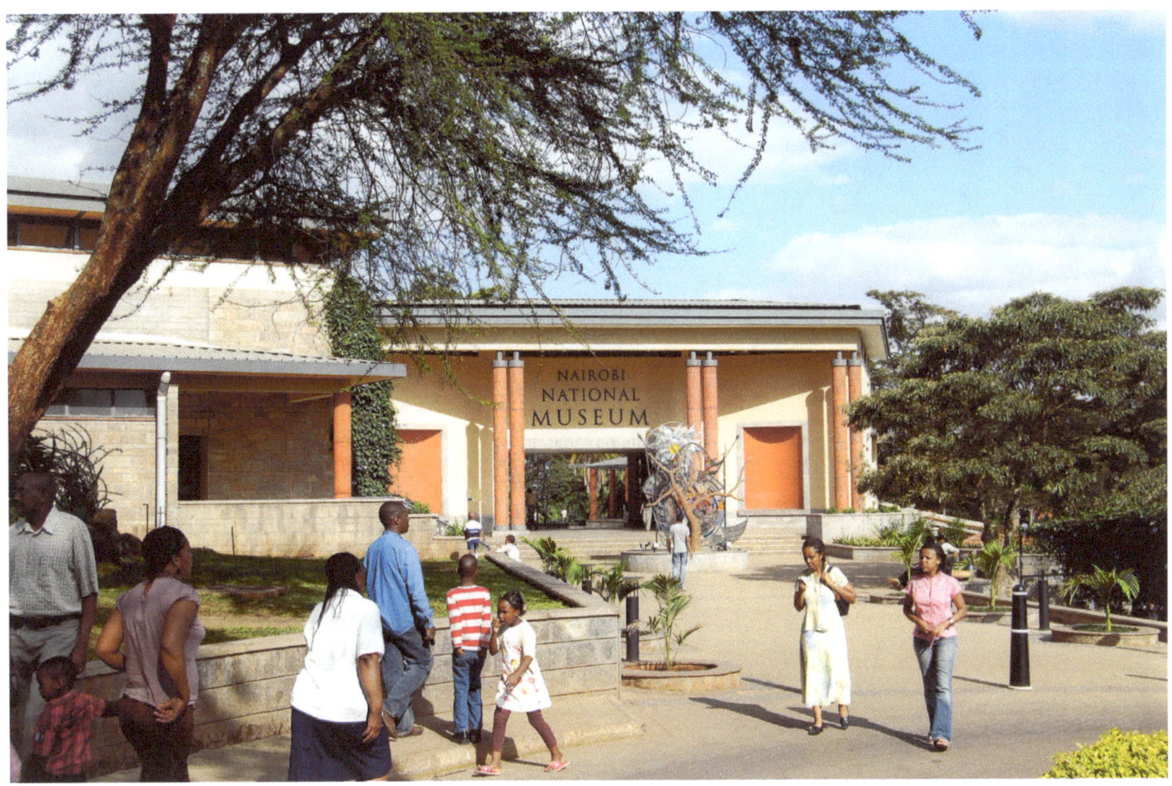

Nairobi Museum.

Guess where we had lunch? You guessed it - Nairobi Java! They love us there. I write love notes to them on the comment cards they provide. I guess they aren't used to having people fill them out as they appeared very concerned and asked Margaret what I wrote. We also heard from Ken Okoth. Ken is a friend from Georgetown and a Kenyan who lives with his family in Kibera during the summer and teaches at Potomac School, and as an adjunct faculty member in Georgetown's School of Foreign Service, during the academic year. He is also the founder of the Children of Kibera Foundation. We will dine with him on Tuesday.

Franco, our newest "best friend and driver," took us on a tour of the city and to the Nairobi National Museum. It was great. Apparently Sunday is the best day to do this since there is very little traffic downtown. What a great city with fascinating economics and class dynamics. At least the roads in downtown Nairobi are nice. You can't say that about many of the roads elsewhere.

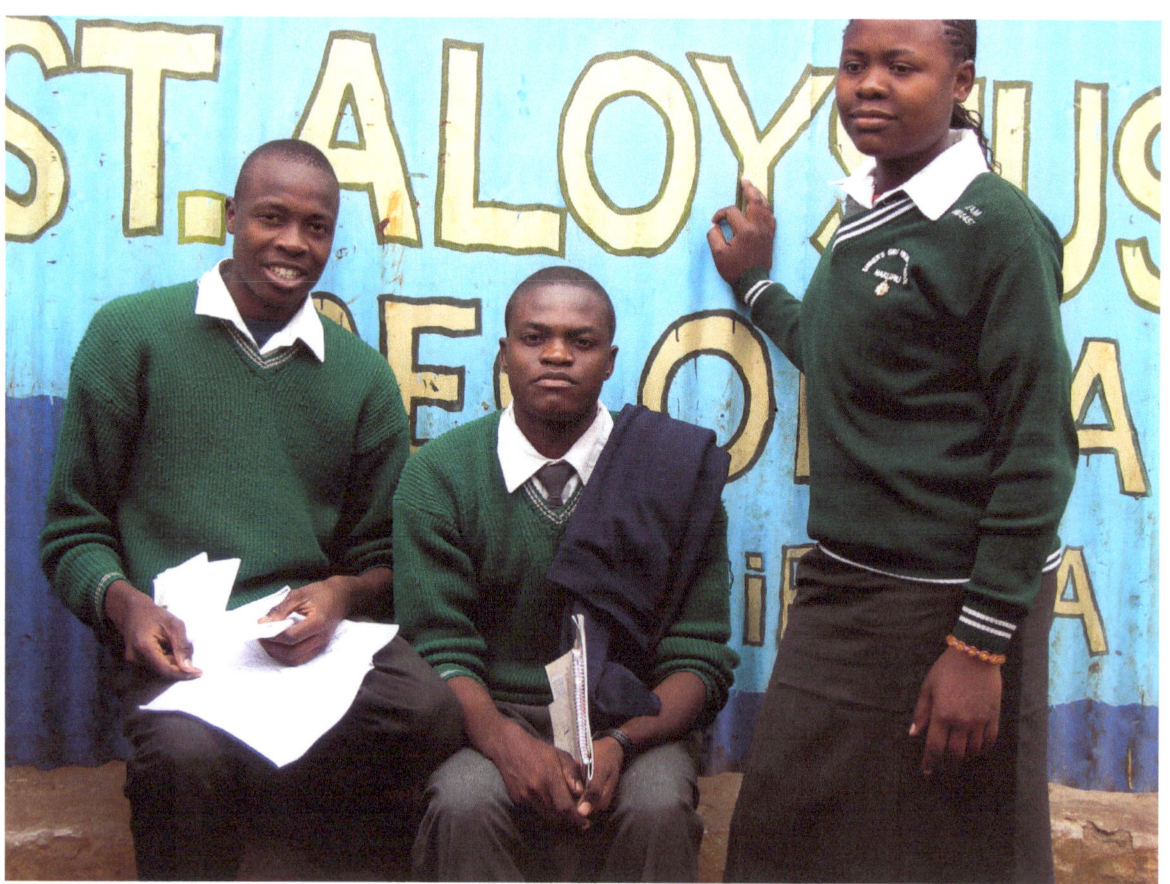

Students at St. Al's.

Surprise, surprise, we ended up back at Nairobi Java for dinner. Yet again, this was another great meal. We will be able to recite the menu for you by the end of this trip.

Today, Monday, was a day of interesting encounters. We went to the Text Book Centre to purchase supplies before class. It feels good to be contributing to the economy here. After getting most of what we needed, we had lunch at Dorman's (Kenya's Starbucks). Great Kenya coffee and good food; sorry, Nairobi Java, but variety is necessary.

Next we went to the school, as planned, to confirm that we'd be teaching at 10am only to learn that we would not be teaching until 2pm. As our dear friend Fr. Phil Boroughs (Vice President for Mission and Ministry at Georgetown University) has said of St. Al's and Kibera, "whatever you planned for, be sure it will be different."

Generally speaking, the students seem excited. Overall, I'd have to say that Form 1 (9th graders) is not as engaged as Form 2 (10th graders). Some of the Form 2 class remembers us from our visit last year. We are teaching them in a style that is very different from what they are used to. We are asking them to engage and respond to us directly. They are accustomed to lectures; the basic mode of education here is read, write and recite.

I think that Margaret and I are great teaching partners – one picks up where the other left off. But after two classes of 35 students each we were positively exhausted!

Tomorrow we start Studio and Class instruction. This is exciting.

After teaching, we went back to Nakumatt Junction for more stuff: Kazuri beads, more supplies and more tea. (Boy, the tea here is great.) After getting the laptop, we are back with our friends at Nairobi Java for dinner and blogging.

We can tell this will be a great experience for us because thus far it has been wonderful.

Charles and Margaret

TUESDAY, AUGUST 12, 2008

We are lucky humans to be experiencing Nairobi in this way.

The Savelberg retreat house is a delightful setting run by the nuns of St. Johns and, boy, oh boy, do they run it. Breakfast at 8 am sharp, tea at 10:30 am on the dot, lunch on your own, and dinner promptly at 7 pm. We haven't experienced dinner here yet - mainly because of me. It's hard for me to imagine dinner anywhere but Nairobi Java - have I mentioned that it's the greatest place on earth, or, at least in

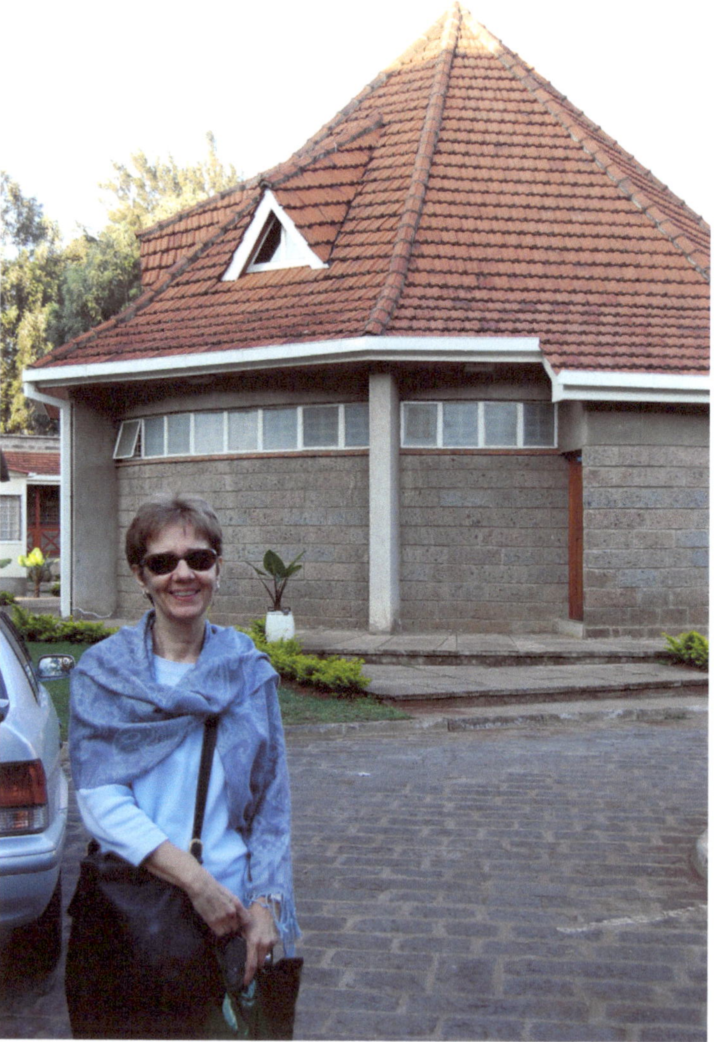

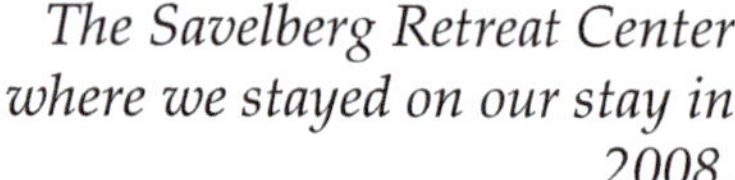

The Savelberg Retreat Center where we stayed on our stay in 2008.

Nairobi? It is also within walking distance of the retreat house. I have been there three times today. At breakfast for fruit, then Margaret and I met our friend, Ken, there for lunch, and again for evening tea before heading out to enjoy dinner with Ken and his fantastic (and large) family in what is called the Olympia neighborhood of Kibera.

Unlike some of the homes we've visited in the past, this was a nice two-bedroom apartment, with a private toilet just for the family. Ken's brother, Jeff, is a culinary school graduate and prepared a fantastic meal of lentils, a delicious beef stew, wonderful homemade chapatti bread, salad, and fresh fruit for dessert. It was absolutely lovely. Ken's mom, Angeline, was amazing and warm and welcoming. Under her stylish shawl she wore an 'Obama for President' shirt. I loved it. If I can figure out how to upload photos to the blog, you may see some pictures of this soon. I also enjoyed Ken's youngest niece who was adorable. She, Angelina, and I are fast friends.

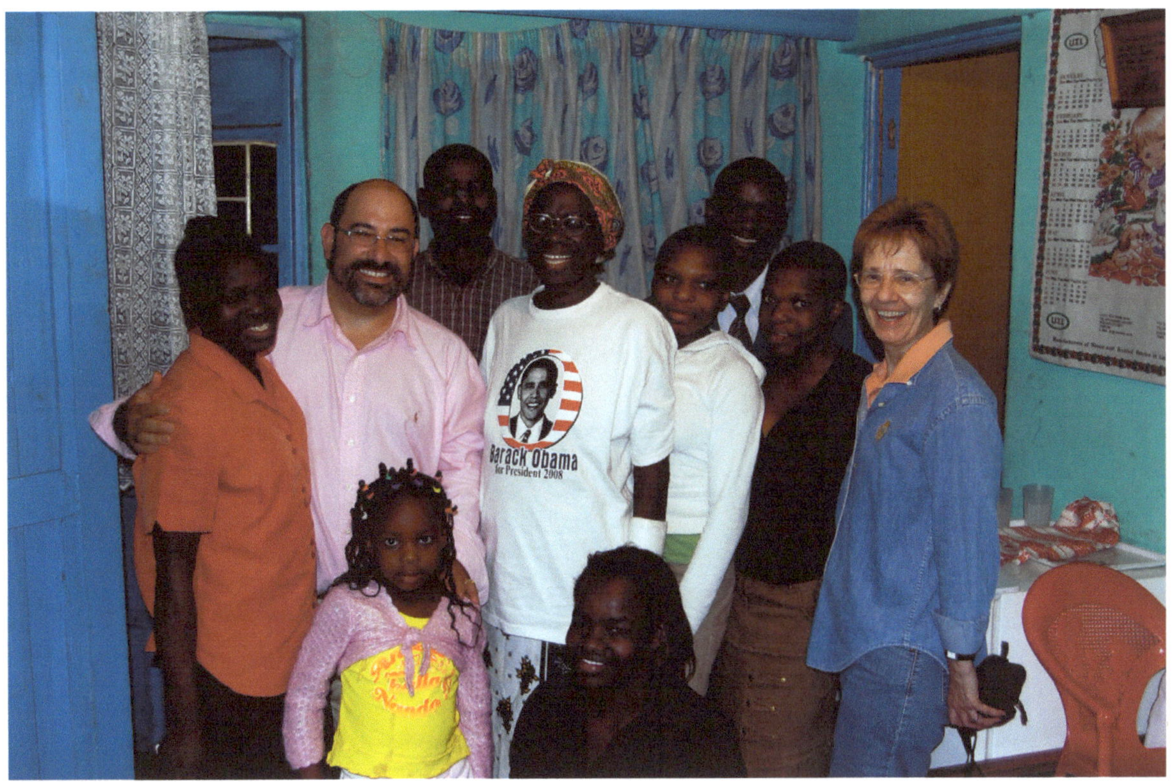

Our visit with Ken Okoth and his family.

Ken and his wife, Monica, spend about six weeks in Nairobi each summer. Monica's family has retired here from Florence, Italy and they live in an area called Lavington, what I consider the high rent district of Nairobi. We joined them at their beautiful estate-like home for a nice glass of wine before we were off to dine with Ken's family. I am struck time and again by the stark contrasts that exist here in Nairobi: retirees from Italy, residents of Kibera. All of which provide a tangible experience of the many types of diversity that co-exist here. Monica's mother, Madeleine, owns a bag shop in Adams Arcade which is located next to Nairobi Java. Wow, they are beautiful bags. Margaret walked into the store and the first thing out of her mouth was "you can never have too many bags." From her mouth to God's ears...and just what the proprietor of a bag shop likes to hear.

Well, all that aside, the meat of our day was spent teaching; a really great experience. It went quickly and intensely today. Yesterday, we posed the question, "what does art mean to you?" The Form 1 class could not answer this question

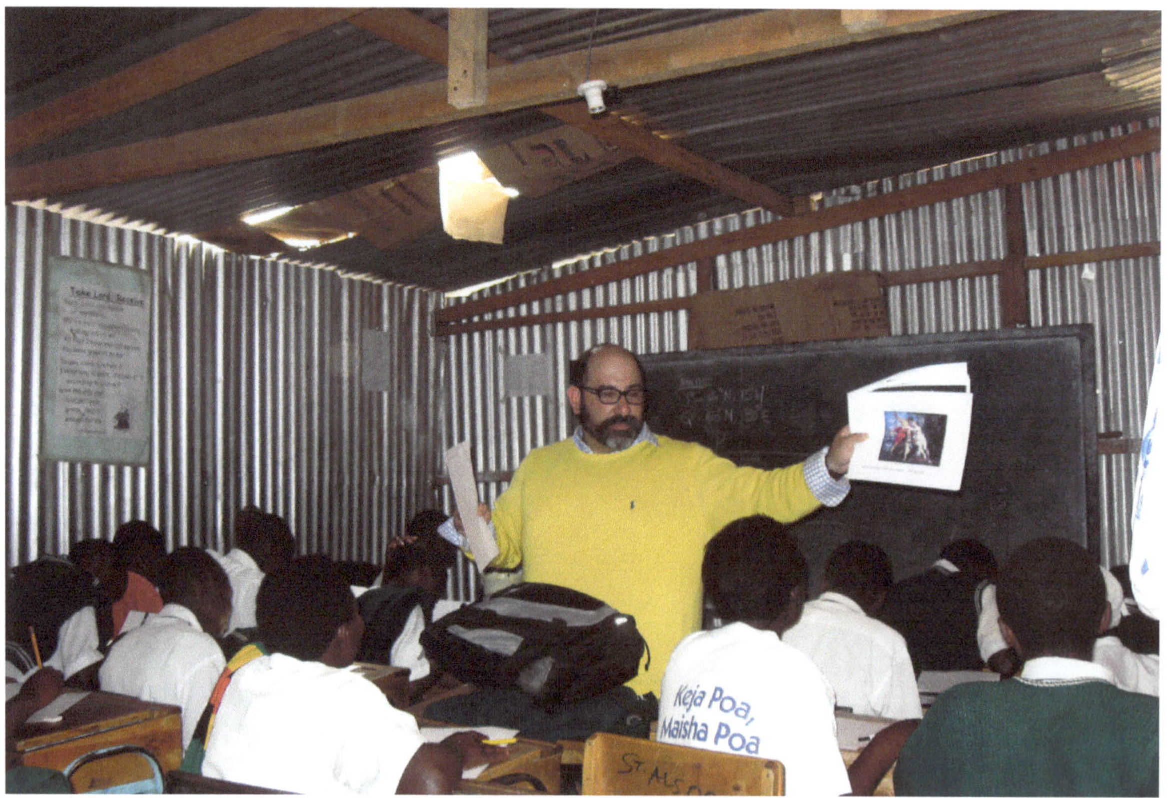

Charles leading an art history lesson at St. Al's.

quickly enough. They came prepared. We introduced Leonardo DaVinci - not DiCaprio, which is what I kept wanting to say - and his Mona Lisa, Renoir and his Boating Party and Toulouse Lautrec and his Moulin Rouge. The students were engrossed. Their homework was to read up on artists and be prepared to answer questions about those artists in class. We also introduced drawing and appointed 'Vice Presidents' in charge of the black and color pencils. These leaders are responsible for the distribution and collection of said pencils to ensure that they will last the full two-week duration of our class. Accountability is a good thing and I am excited to see what comes of it.

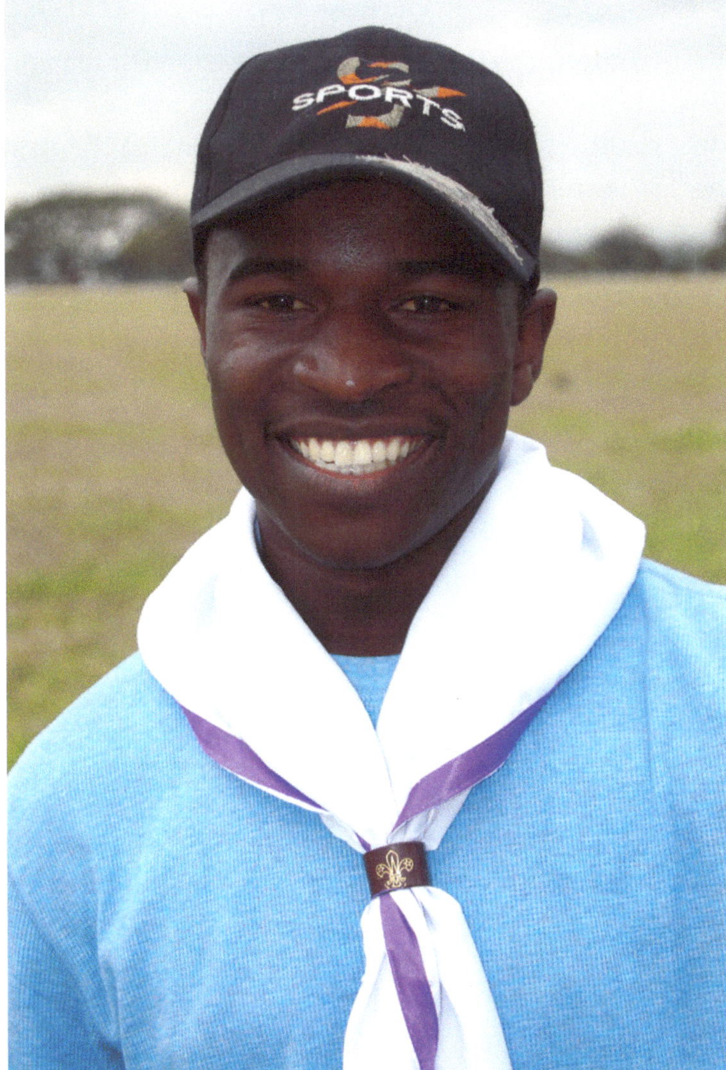

David Dinda.

Today we also started studio sessions. After class with Form 1, they had studio time to work on two assignments: drawing a figure of choice and drawing something from imagination. Wow, I almost had to tear the paper out of their hands to get them to stop at the end of the session. Since they knew Renoir and Lautrec were French, I threw in a few French words and it was downhill from there. *En Chante, Je m'appelle (insert name), Au Revoir.* I had no idea we would be combining French and Art. It made me wish I knew more French.

Margaret and I were running back and forth between classes once studio time started and the other class was simultaneously in session. It was great, feverish and hard work. With 35 students in each class, there is a lot to be done. Margaret and I complement each other well in this setting: I am loud and dramatic, she is calm and reassuring. Her twelve years of experience in the classroom show up clearly as she is an expert teacher; my strengths show up in my passion for art and educating others. Not to toot our own horns, but I think we are working out well.

After class today, David Dinda stopped by to say hello. He is one of the first graduates of St. Al's. Two colleagues of mine from Georgetown, Lynne Hirshfeld and Lyndon Dominique, and I supported him pursuing Social Work College. I've connected with him in a powerful way; he feels like a son to me. I look forward to spending more time with him while we're here.

So, after dinner and the whole day of it all, Margaret and I are simultaneously exhausted and bouncing off the ceilings; bed is the farthest thing from our minds.

More to come.... It only gets more exciting and a bit overwhelming with all the contrasts we continue to encounter. From wine at an estate to a wonderful family dinner in the largest slum on the continent of Africa, it all represents Kenya.

Charles and Margaret

WEDNESDAY, AUGUST 13, 2008
Teaching and Scouting. What????

Today was yet another amazing day. We visited the Red Rose School, a primary school in Kibera created by the Children of Kibera Foundation, to see the children in session. The kids are amazing and very excited about learning. Margaret and I are going to be working there a few mornings next week. The one thing I have to say is – in case I haven't said it already – teaching is hard work. I cannot imagine teaching eight classes a day, five days a week. It's overwhelming the amount of preparation, attention and patience required.

We had lunch at Nairobi Java and then we headed to St. Al's. We had a productive day and now most of our lecture curriculum has been covered. The students

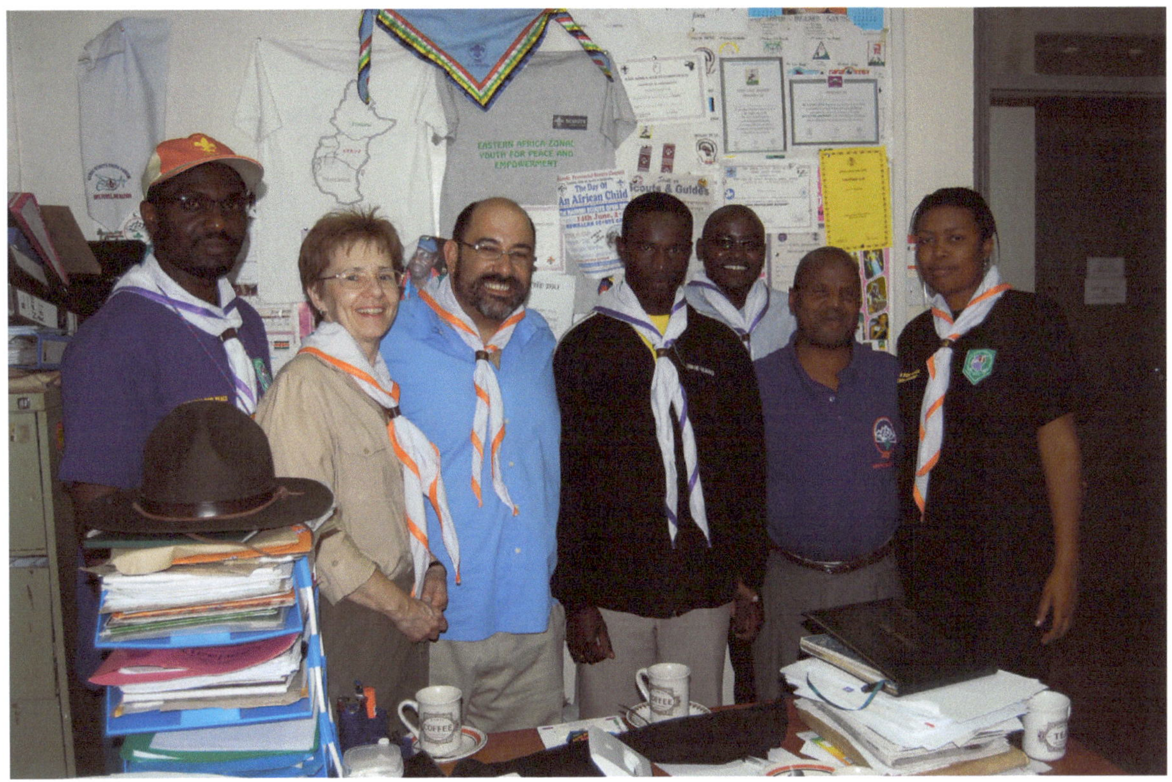

We are inducted as honorary Rovers into the Kenya Scouts.

have really clicked with the artists and art works that we've shared and they are getting it. Forty students over the next week will be asked to tell the class about the "top 20" well-known western artists. Two students are in the process of researching Socrates as a result of our sharing the painting Death of Socrates by David with them.

We're now moving into studio mode. The kids continue to do really well with drawing. Tomorrow they'll begin painting.

Okay. Scouting. On the road into Kibera, there is a Kenyan Scout Center. The founder of the Scouts in the US also started the Scouts here. He loved Kenya so much that he wanted to be buried here, and, so, he rests in Nyeri.

Well, as a boy, I was a Scout. My scouting career, however, was brief. I only made it to Star. Margaret was a Girl Scout and it shows - she is definitely a more prepared person. So yesterday I said to Franco, "Do you think we can stop at the Scout Center so I can get a badge that says Nairobi?," We did and…oh. My. God.

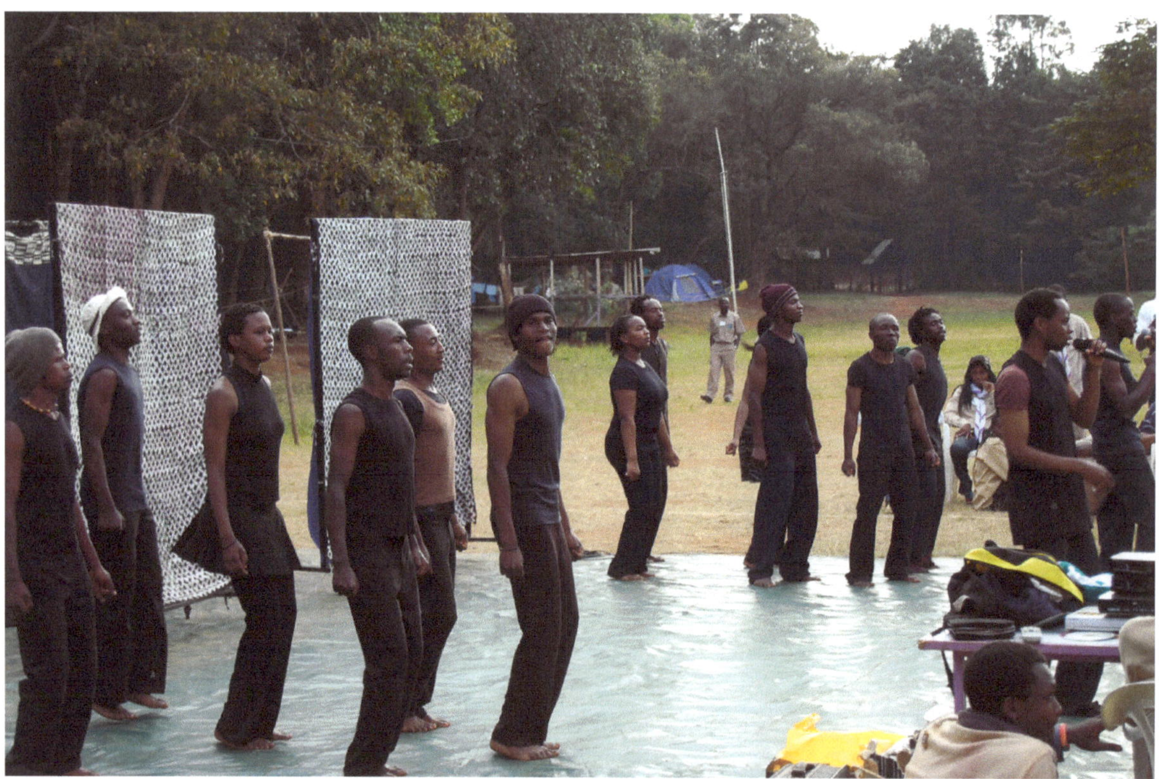

Performance troupe focuses on HIV and AIDS-awareness and prevention themes at Kenyan Scouting event.

As it turns out, it is Moot Scout Week during which all of the East African Scouts come together to practice scouting and other related activities. The Kenyan Scouts include both boys and girls; they do not have a separate organization based on gender as we do in the States. So, the Director in Nairobi and the Special Programme Commissioner for the Scouts happened to be there when I walked in and asked for a badge. The rest is history. The Director and the Commissioner were so impressed that we would stop by that they pulled together an on-the-spot ceremony to bestow upon us the highest honor possible for adult scouts, induction into The Rovers. With cameras and video recorders rolling, Margaret and I were presented with scarves in ceremonial fashion, Franco and David were made World Scouts, and we all got badges and were presented to the entire camp. I was in shock. All I wanted was a couple of badges that said Nairobi. We are official Kenyan Scouts! The Scouts have asked us to come back anytime. I can't believe our luck that we are now a part of this wonderful organization that does outreach and education on many important topics ranging from organic agriculture, AIDS education, and equality - just to name a few. While we were there, HIV testing was being done and a magnet theatre group was performing to promote AIDS/HIV-awareness and to break down the myths and misconceptions about the disease; so impressive. Little did I suspect when I woke up this morning that by the end of the day Margaret and I would belong to the Kenyan Scouts. Just another day in Nairobi.

I hope all is well and I will write again tomorrow.

Charles and Margaret

THURSDAY, AUGUST 14, 2008
Day 5 of teaching. Can you believe it???

Time is flying and, I have to say, it is wonderful. Now that we've been inducted into the Kenyan Scouts as Rovers, it's all downhill from here!

Yesterday it was nice to have David Dinda spend the morning with us as we ran some errands to prepare for class. Then Franco suggested we see the interior of the old Norfolk Hotel. This hotel was given to Kenya as a Christmas present in 1904 by Major C.G.R. Ringer. It is amazing and has been completely renovated. What a treat. The coffee was amazing, the gift shop was very high–end. Then off to lunch at Nairobi Java and to school for another speedy and wonderful day.

Although we may appear to be teaching just two hours, we're actually teaching two distinct classes simultaneously. Yesterday was more studio time along with

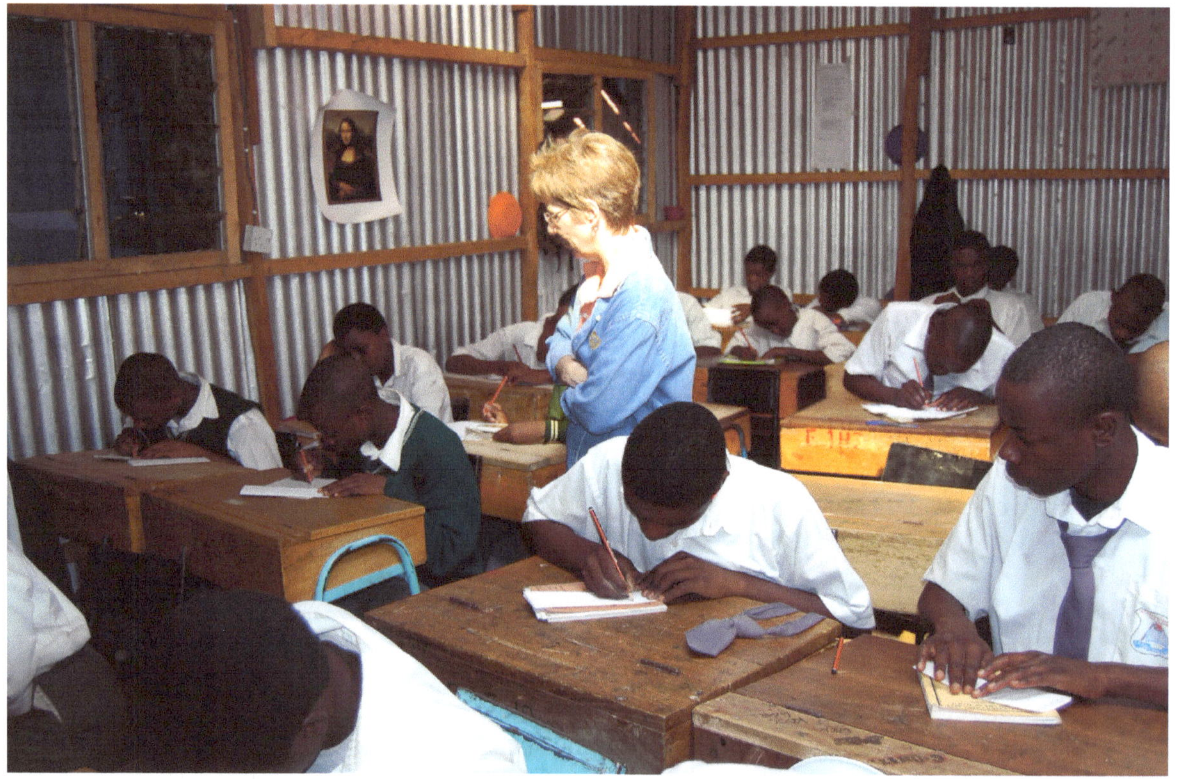

Margaret Halpin provides instruction during studio session.

student readings of artists' biographies. We love hearing them read aloud so beautifully and can't help but smile when they all ask for copies of the material – there's such an eagerness to learn!

Margaret has the students doing timed drawings while I have them completing their color drawings. Compared to the colored pencils, they don't like black pencils. They love color. It is great to see how well they are doing. They are all amazing humans filled with so much potential.

Headmaster Kiambi came by and told us how happy he is with the program. So happy, in fact, that we are planning dates for 2009. I could not be more thrilled to know that the school has invited us back.

At the end of the day we handed out cameras to five team leaders who are tasked with taking pictures of their lives and the lives of their assigned groups. I cannot wait to see what we get.

The children respond well in class, ask questions and take true responsibility. They are protective of this art immersion in a way that I would not have imagined. We wanted to leave the art posters that we brought and were going to put them up in the classroom but they said, "No, we want them to stay safe, clean and cared for; put them in the library."

Although Margaret and I are giving our time, knowledge and skills, we are really receiving so much more from these beautiful and smart students. One student, who was tasked with researching Socrates, came to me upset because all she could find about him was that he was a Greek philosopher. And yet she was able to discover that much with extremely limited access and resources! They are equally engaged on all fronts.

Well, believe it or not, after today only one week of teaching remains. We are shocked that it has gone so quickly, and we have so much to do...

Much love and we miss you all,

Charles and Margaret

FRIDAY, AUGUST 15, 2008
First week down. What amazing students.

Although we had a general idea of what this art immersion program would be, we really didn't know what to expect. These students have most certainly blown any expectations we may have had totally out of the water. Every day I tell the students that they are smart, beautiful and important. They are that – and then some.

Their drawings are hard to comprehend. Particularly when you realize they've never been exposed to art, have never had anything remotely like this experience, and then see how some of them so get what we've been working on. You look at some of these drawings and think, "Wow, they made Kibera beautiful. It looks beautiful." Margaret has really been able to focus the students on the importance of genre, form and landscape. They all get it.

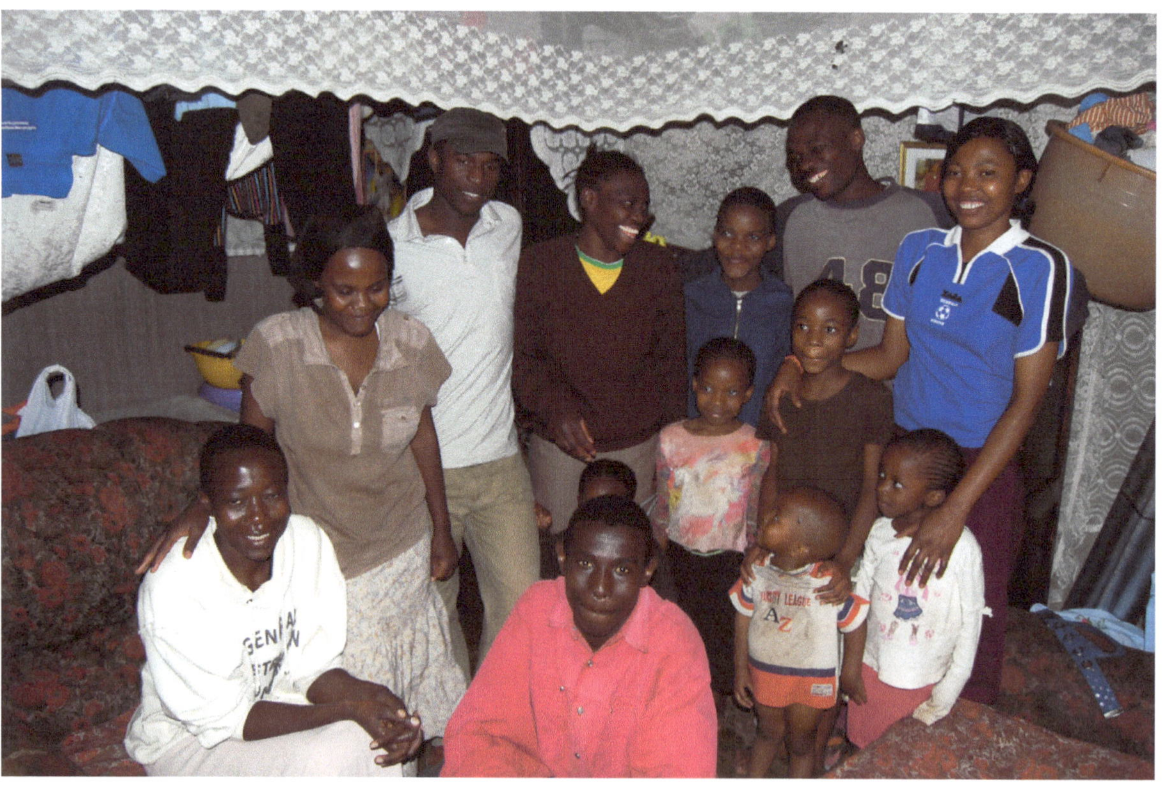

Visiting the home of David Dinda's brother in Kibera.

I love hearing them read about history and pronounce Toulouse Lautrec in their Kenyan Swahili British accent; they are so proud when they are asked to speak in front of the class.

I think we've been most impressed with their photography. As we look at what they've begun to submit, we keep asking each other "Did they take that?" Wow. The pictures are so beautiful, hard, and revealing - not what we expected from their first 24 hours with the cameras. They have the cameras for the weekend and I cannot wait to see what they come up with on Monday.

After class we went to David Dinda's brother's home where we met four siblings, five nieces/nephews and many other people. Seven people live in a single 7′ x 7′ room. David also showed us his home where he lives on his own so he can study. It is small with no water, although electricity is rigged in somehow.

We saw inner Kibera and it was filled with squalor, beauty, hope, pain, abject poverty and, at the same time, it is a welcoming place. As I've said before, the most alarming aspects of Nairobi are the contrasts. We spent the morning in Muthaiga in the village market. This is by far the highest socio-economic district of Nairobi, Kenya, with nice stores and an open air market, as well as a great chocolate shop (you know me). In the markets, Margaret and I established our own shopping protocol. She would find something she wanted and I'd come in for the kill, bargaining until we got what we wanted. If that didn't work, I would walk away, wait awhile and then circle back.

At the end of the day, after looking at our emerging art and photography projects with Deputy Headmistress Beatrice, she asked me how many years Margaret and I had been teaching in this type of setting. I must admit that her question made me nervous because I wasn't sure what she was going to say. Luckily, she said that she could never have imagined that the students would be this talented and demonstrate it in such a short time. She was so excited to see the beauty in their work and the talent they exhibit. Wouldn't it be great to see one of these students having their work on display in a museum? One never knows! Anything is possible.

More later,

Charles and Margaret

MONDAY, AUGUST 18, 2008

More than Art. A weekend and the start of week 2.

After Saturday morning at the Mikono Shop at the Jesuit Refugee Services in Nairobi, we attempted to see the orphaned elephants at the Sheldrick Center in Langata. We discovered that viewing was allowed only one hour each day, so we went back to Savelberg (home sweet home) for an afternoon rest before picking up my dear friend, Anne Wangari to have dinner with Father Superior of East Africa, Valerian Shirima.

Dinner was so great and so was the company. We had a lovely meal and a great time with wonderful, witty and caring conversation.

Sunday was a packed day. Margaret went to a church she had been wanting to visit and Mass lasted about 45 minutes longer than she expected. Then we went

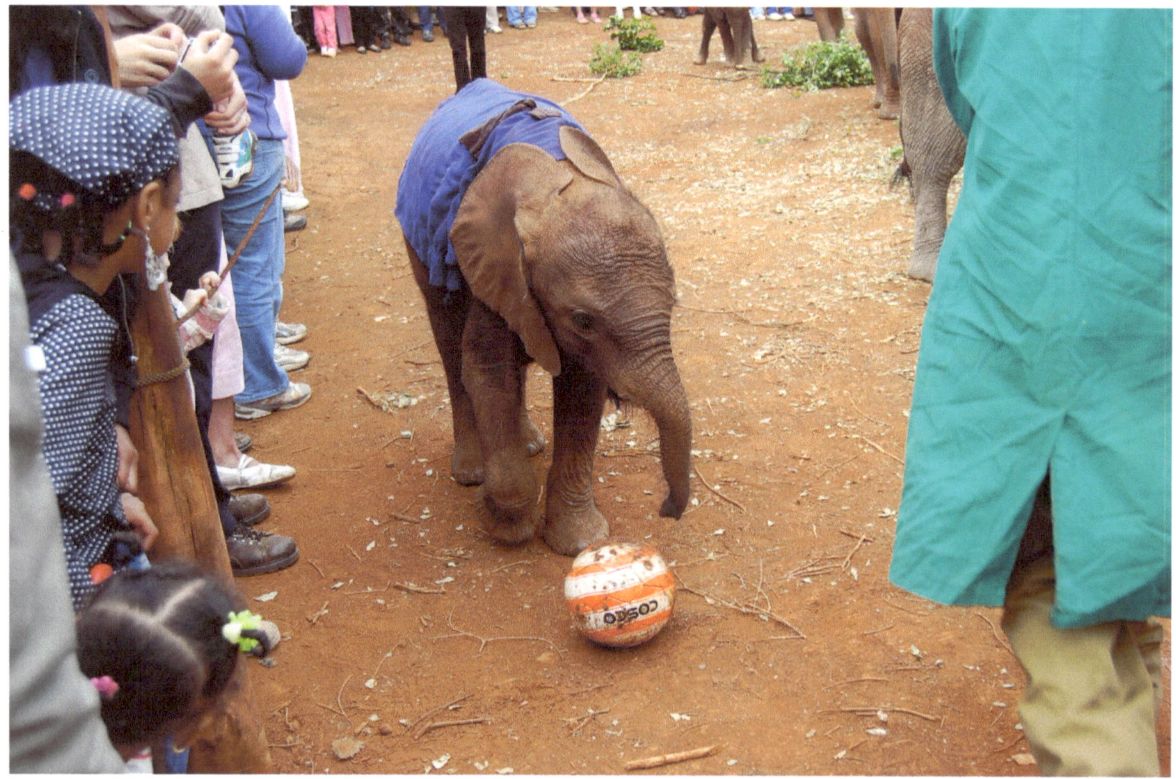

A young orphaned elephant puts on a show.

again to see the elephants. On this occasion we timed it well—we actually saw them! - and it was great. There were ten elephants ranging from 2- to 23-months old. They'd been orphaned for reasons ranging from human impact to natural causes. I took about 500 pictures. Elephants are my new favorite animal; they've always been Margaret's favorite. After our date with the elephants, we were off to the Verandah for eating and shopping (at least looking).

Next, we visited with Deborah Moijoi from Pedro Arrupe. We picked up Deborah and Father Toppo, who is a retired Jesuit in residence at Pedro Arrupe, and headed to her house to see her family and have tea. Delightful.

Off to dinner at Nakumatt Juntion at Nairobi Java. Have I mentioned that we love this place? We ate with Anne Wangari and had a really wonderful time.

Now we are starting our second and final week of the St. Al's Art Immersion Program. We kicked things off with an introduction to watercolor and then had Forms 1 and 2 try it for themselves. It is so amazing to see these kids learning so

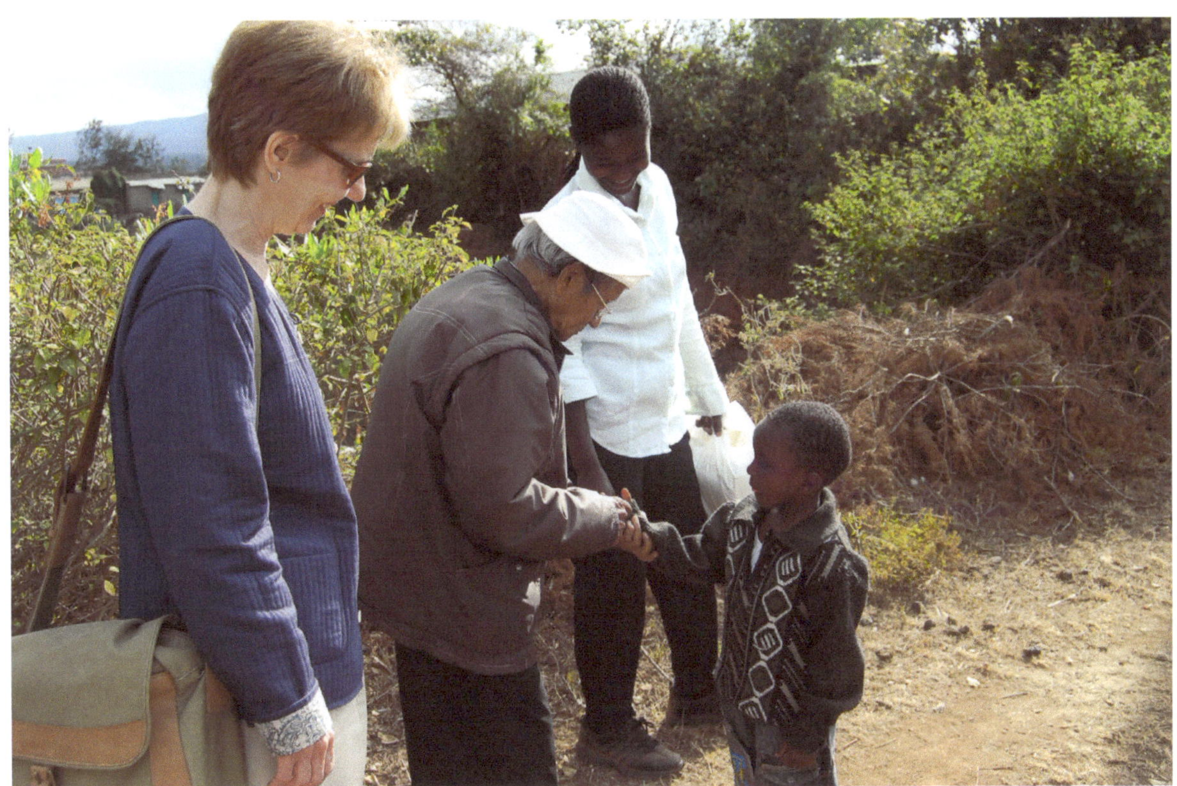

Margaret and Fr. Toppo with Debora Moijoi and her nephew.

quickly and producing such great art. We also got the cameras back today. The photos that these kids are taking truly tell a story. I am so thrilled that we will be able to share this with you. These young people have a stock pile of hidden talents. I feel like we could spend day after day with them and never have enough time. Tonight we dine with Sr. Mary Owens of Nyumbani. We are so fortunate to have these connections here and are so humbled by how gracious everyone has been in connecting with us while we are here.

We will keep you up to date on our progress. Thanks for all your interest and support.

Charles and Margaret

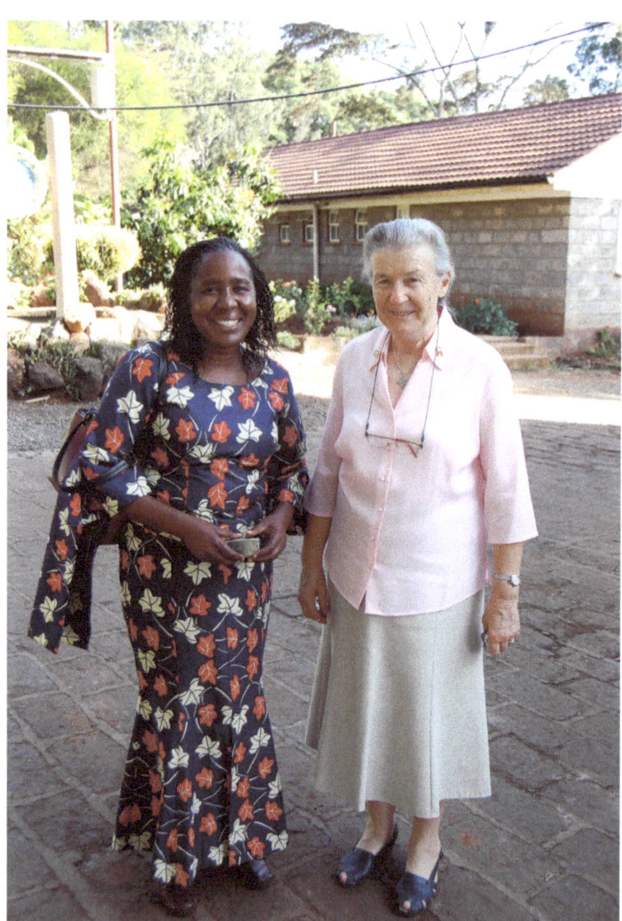

Anne Wangari and Sr. Mary Owen.

TUESDAY, AUGUST 19, 2008
Harsh realities show up on week 2, day 2.

This morning I wasn't feeling well due to sinus stuff and some dehydration. I am, however, recovered. Besides, there's no rest for the weary; we were off to St. Al's to prepare to teach more watercolors. Once there, the harsh realities of daily life in Kibera showed up. In preparation for our studio work with water colors, we asked our students to get water for their painting. They came back and informed us that the water had been shut off for rationing. Wow. Can you imagine coming home and not being able to use your water or any of the other resources we don't think twice about? It is just a shocker. Take that to the next level and realize that one of the only places in Kibera where these students have access to running water is at the school.

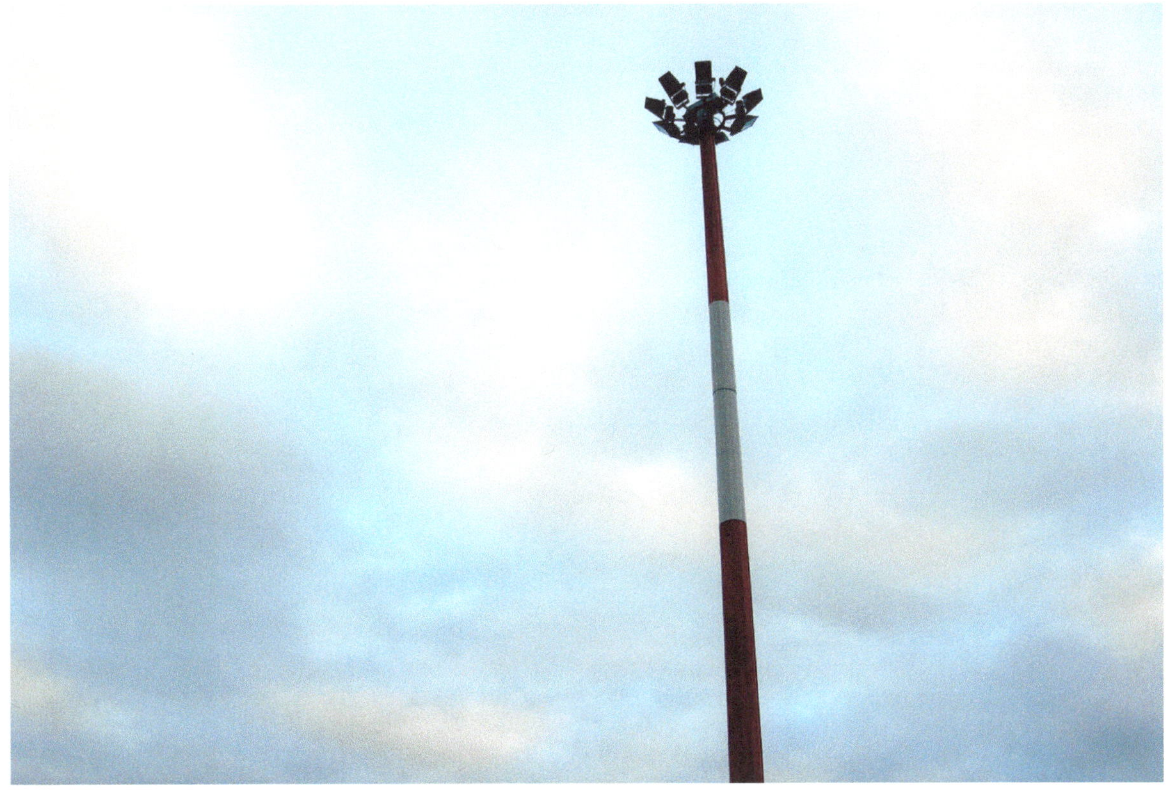

Student photo taken in Kibera.

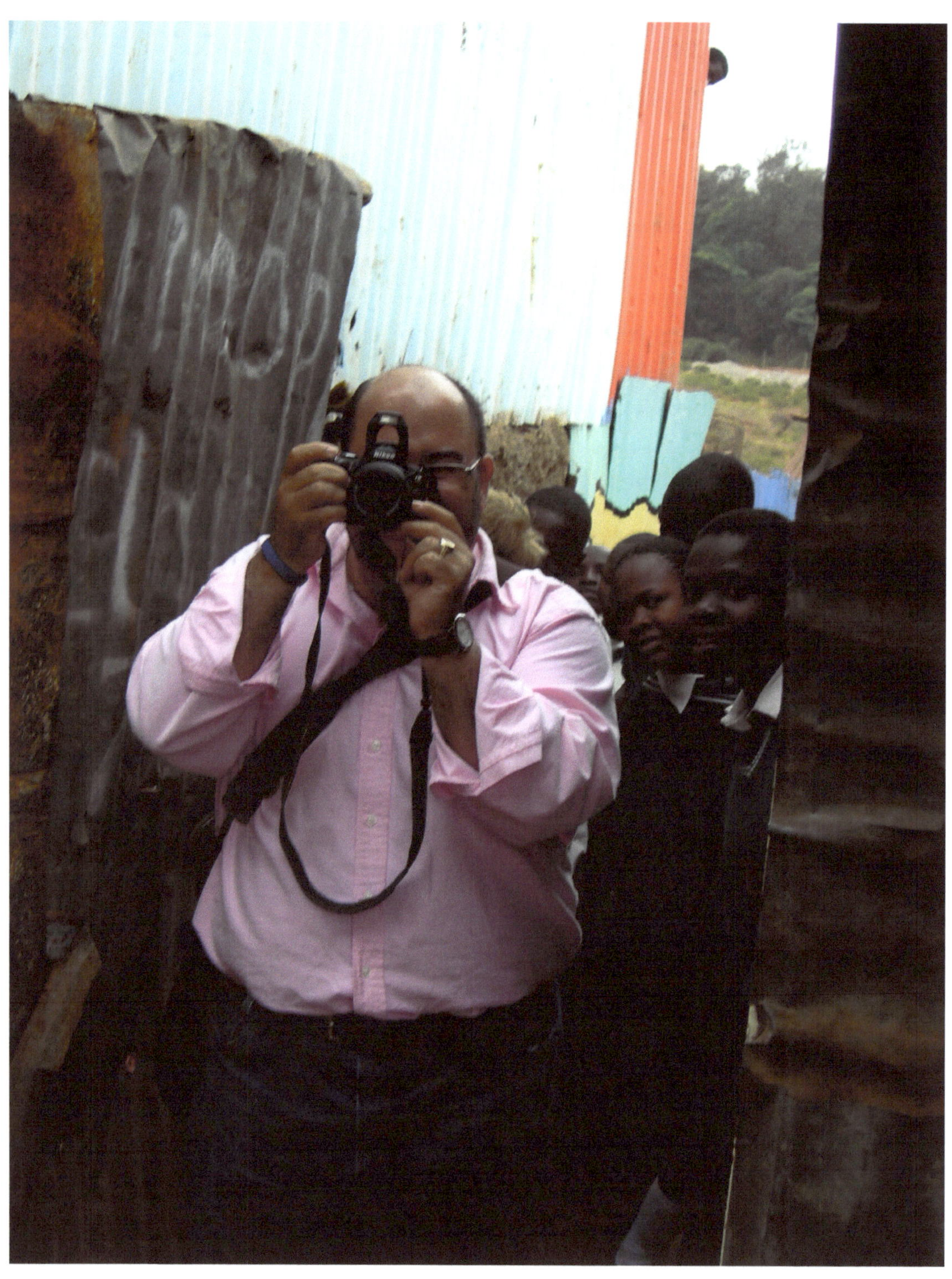

Student photo taken in Kibera.

When faced with a situation like this you just roll with it. After last week, Margaret and I each settled with a class: Margaret has Form 1 and I have Form 2. The first week we were co-teaching but now we have each settled into a groove that makes sense. Occasionally we end up popping into each other's classes and it works really well.

Yesterday we had the students create an artists' biography for themselves. Reading them just made our hearts stop; so few words with so much meaning. They are so intent on succeeding that all you want to do is help pave the road. Their lives are hard and yet they pull it together in school, hope for the best and readily acknowledge that there are others who are worse off.

Since we didn't have water for paints, Margaret's class drew and my class continued the "top 20" history curriculum. They love the top 20 and often when those that have volunteered to read are asked to, we have to collect the reading material from someone else who wanted to read it outside of class. It makes you realize how hungry they are for knowledge. These students are smart.

Last night Margaret and I looked at over 1000 photographs that these kids have already taken. We are in awe of the stories these pictures tell. We also have many minutes of video that were captured when the kids realized they could do it.

The paintings and drawings are also great and so expressive. The other night when we met with Sr. Mary Owens, she told us that the kids don't have opportunities to express themselves and that, she believed, this must be so freeing for them.

I love it. I feel we're getting as much out of this experience, if not more, as the students are.

Thanks for all your support.

Charles and Margaret

WEDNESDAY, AUGUST 20, 2008
Never let water get in the way of painting.

Today is the third day of week two. We created certificates for our 70 students that we'll give out on Friday. These students deserve so much more.

This morning we taught Standards 1 and 2 at the Red Rose School and had them draw animals. They were so well behaved and excited to have us there.

Got to St. Al's only to find, once again, there was no water. But who said it can't come from elsewhere?

In order to paint, volunteers from each class were tasked with going to a place where they knew they could get water and - voila - we were in action. Painting all around. Some of the student's painting skills are very pedestrian since this is,

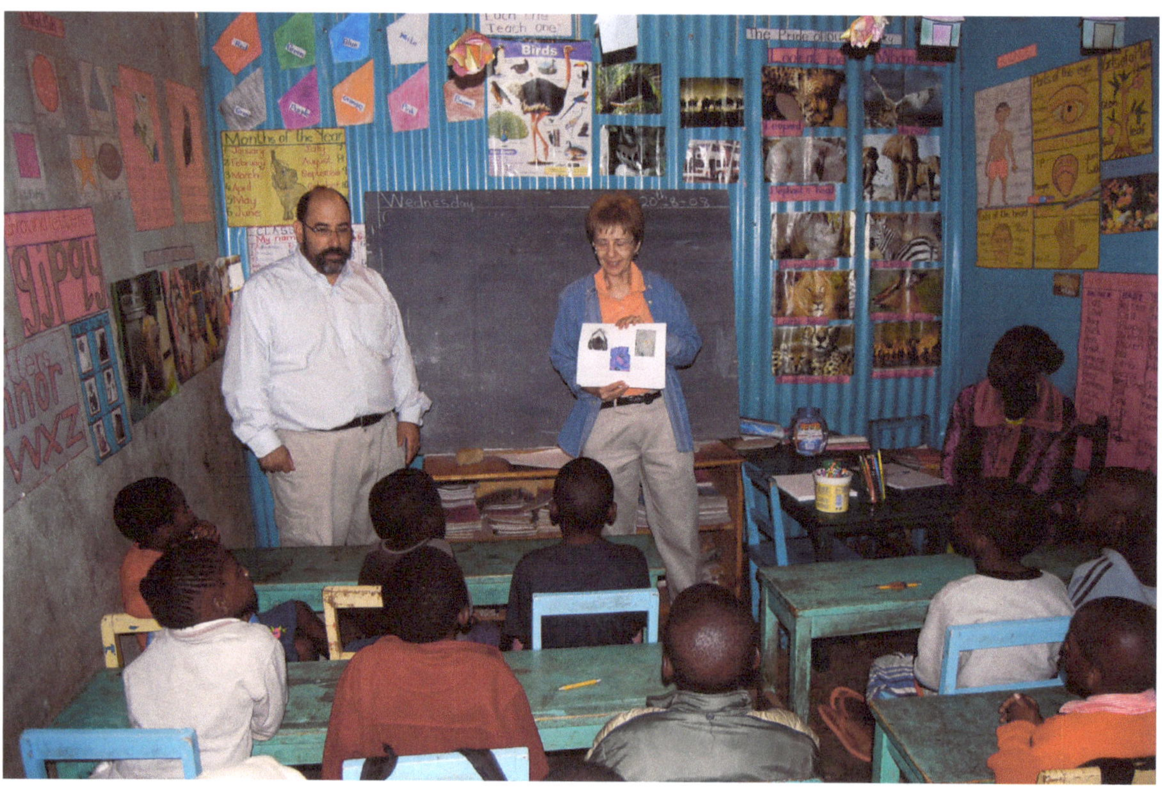

We provide basic art instruction at the Red Rose School.

literally for some, the first time that they've ever painted. Others who have been exposed to drawing and other artistic mediums are doing great. There is one student in particular who should be in a school for the arts or, at least, going to art classes on the side.

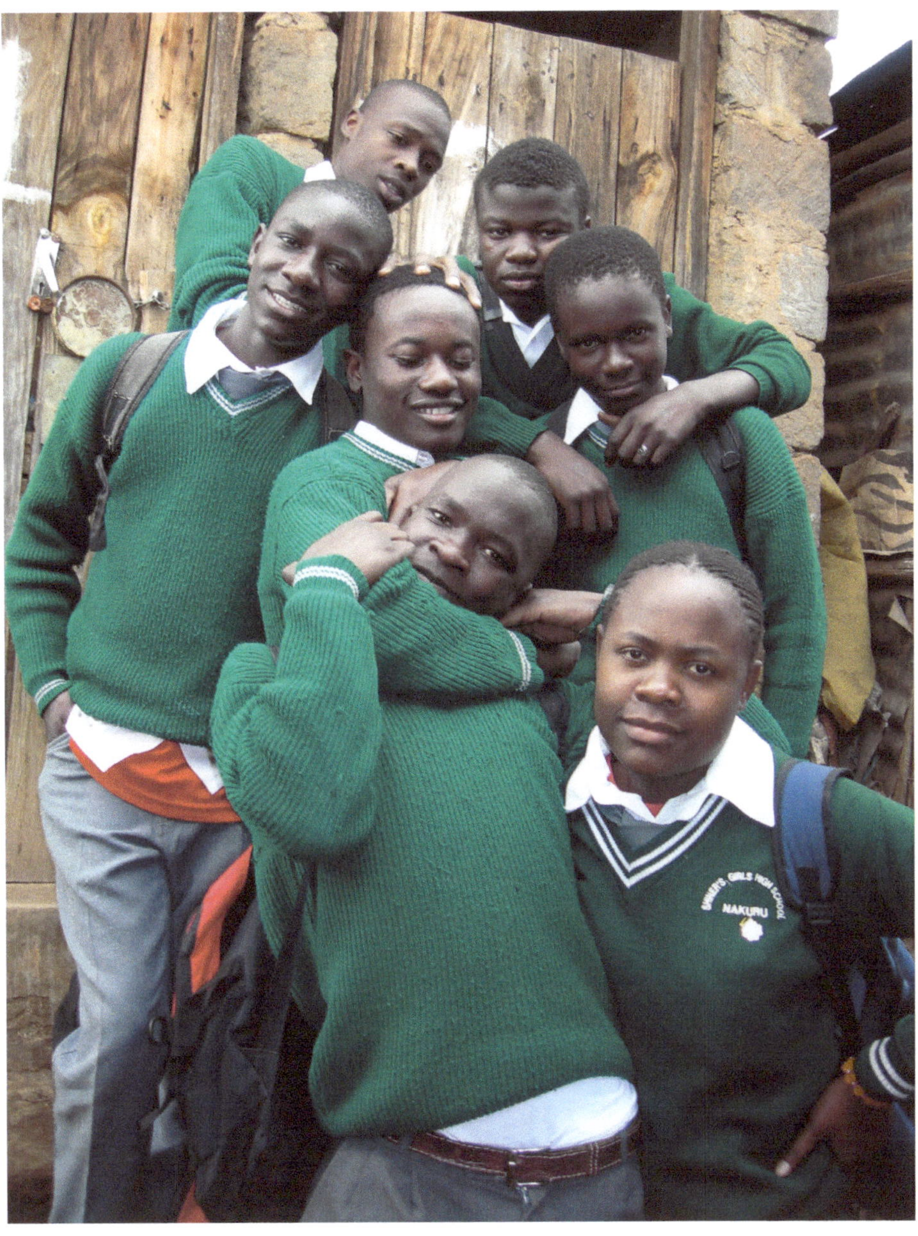

Student photo.

The classes were bustling for the whole two hours. The students seemed like they could continue far beyond the allotted time. Some have endless energy and only a few seem to just be going through the motions of making art. We've heard from other teachers at the school that Forms 1 and 2 seem to only talk about the art classes, which is great. When we're done with this year's program we'll leave some source materials in the library so the kids can continue to look at the biographies of the artists; we'll also encourage them to start an art club of sorts with the materials that we've brought. I am hopeful that they will continue to explore and develop their skills.

All the cameras came back today. As always, they carry interesting stories. At the same time, one must remember that the photographers are teenagers and that perspective certainly comes across in many of the pictures. Who doesn't like posing, right? Well, it seems that we have what seems like thousands of students who were meant to be on the runway. These kids love to have their photo taken.

Tomorrow is the fourth day of week two, and probably the last real day of class since on Friday we'll be giving out certificates and sharing art and photos. Then we go back to our lives of - what I began to consider last year as - abject luxury. Having experienced this second visit to Kenya, now I am sure of it.

After class we were able to visit with Laban Manga, a man we met on our trip last year. Laban runs the small letter presses at St. Joseph, and he and I have stayed in contact throughout the year. Once he learned we were coming this summer he invited us to meet his wife and daughter at his home in Kengami, another slum in Nairobi. It was a nice visit and it made me realize that all slums are not created equal. His home has a true door, a living room, kitchen and, I am sure, a bedroom. There is a distinct difference between Kengami and Kibera. Laban was telling us that in December/January when the riots and fires hit in the wake of the post election violence, he had five people from Kibera living with him. The view from his home was great and, at the same time, it was of Kibera. As we have experienced on this trip, there is a lot of awkward beauty in Nairobi.

That is all for now.

Charles and Margaret

THURSDAY, AUGUST 21, 2008
Third world charm.

Yesterday, the fact that we didn't have running water couldn't prevent us from painting. Today, the fact that we didn't have running water ***or*** power couldn't stop us either. Margaret and I got to the school on time, the students were getting prepared as usual, but when we went into the deputy headmistress' office (which we've been using as our office while we're here) we found her sitting there in the dark holding a meeting with a parent and student as if it was no big deal. I guess you just make the best of it, and that's what we did.

Today was important because it was the day we distributed the good paper for watercolor painting. It was also the last class during which we'll be making art.

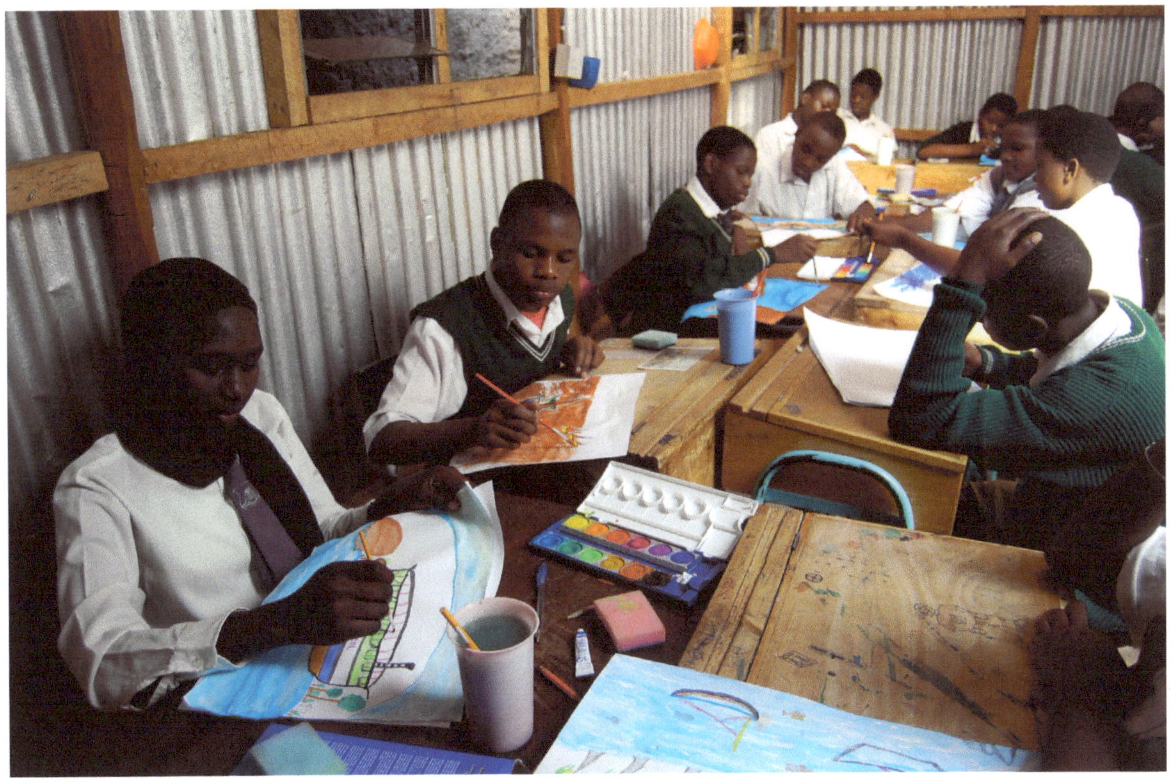

St. Al's students focus on watercolors during studio session.

The history lessons have been deployed, the concepts have been taught and, today, the masterpieces were created. The students were really engaged in their projects. They were supposed to go to gym class at 3 pm but asked if they could paint until the very end of the school day because they wanted to make the most of their time with us. These students are amazing. You see their personalities come through in how they ask questions, express themselves and in how they paint. My Form 2 class is oh so quiet when they're painting. Margaret's freshmen seem to be a little more talkative and well, you know, freshmen.

The patron of the classes that we're teaching is Sr. Luciana. She came by to say how excited she was about this program and that she hoped the work would not stop once we leave. I was delighted to hear her propose that it continue on a weekly basis. Margaret and I will meet with the headmaster tomorrow to discuss how that might happen. Indeed, the kids are abuzz with art.

The Kenyan people are resilient and it shows in how these students persevere and push forward. Their energy and enthusiasm is contagious and makes you

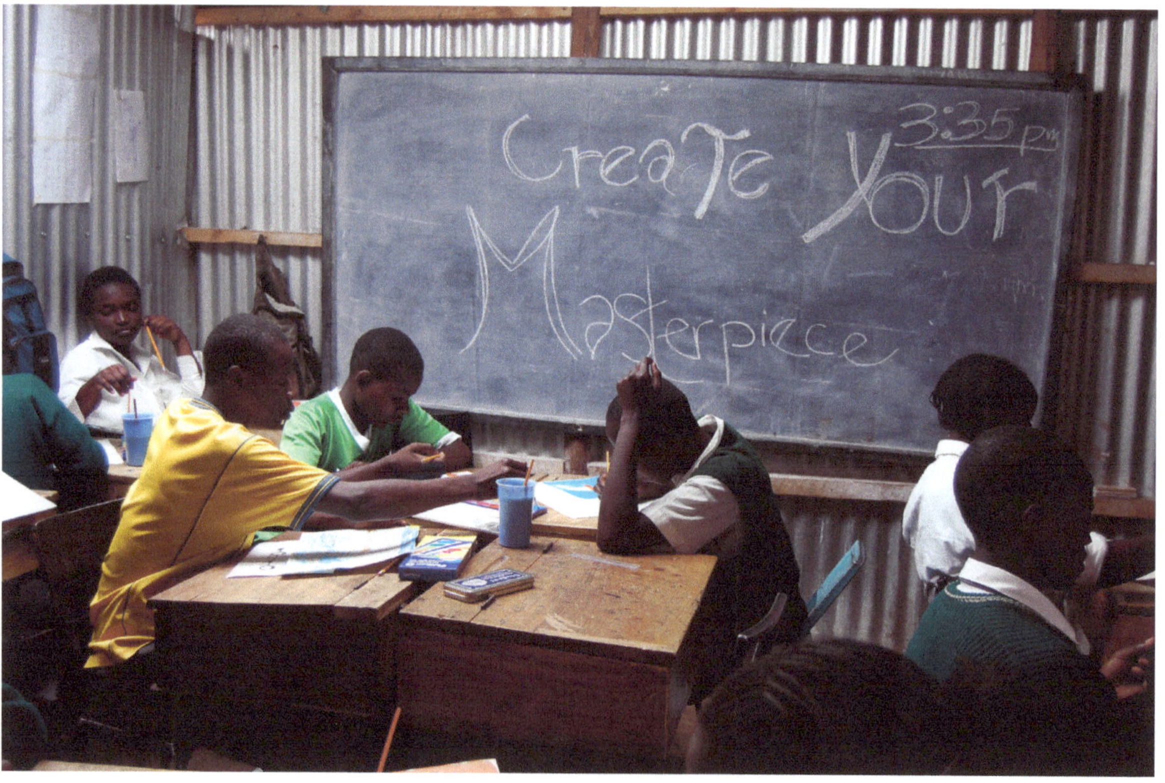

Students contemplate their next masterpiece.

want to do as much as you can with them. They're a loving, engaging and welcoming people.

Thanks to Margaret, St. Al's library will now house posters of great works of art along with two readers that she compiled based on our art history curriculum.

Don't think either of us can believe that tomorrow will be our last day with the students. We're both still settling in to the surroundings and have become attached to Nairobi, Kibera, the people, and our students.

This trip is a catalyst for whatever might be next. Who knows? I told the class that I had a dream of them showing their art in the Nairobi Art Institute. Although no such place exists – yet! - they burst into spontaneous applause and you could see the excitement on their faces reflecting the possibility that this could really happen someday.

As I keep telling them, they are smart, beautiful and important. I've gotten so much more than I've given. We are lucky humans.

Tomorrow we'll head off to Village Market in the morning, pick up some beverages for our celebration at the school and then we'll honor the great artists of St. Al's for their accomplishments. To see them so happy makes you realize that it is all worth it. Every bit of it.

More tomorrow,

Charles and Margaret

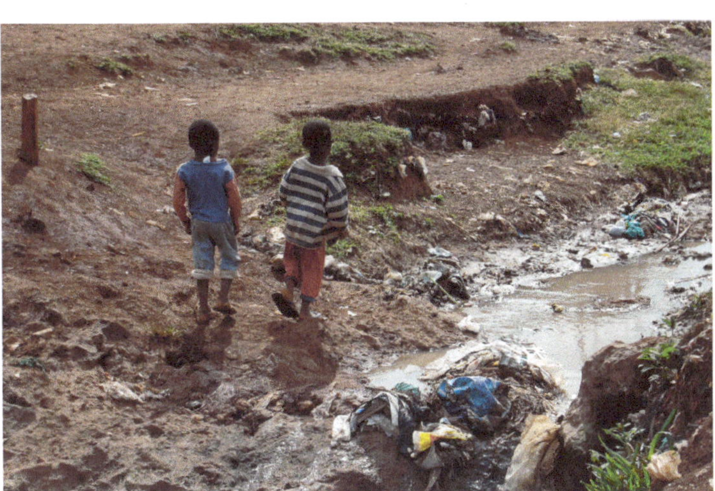

Young residents of the Kibera slum.

FRIDAY, AUGUST 22, 2008
Our last day: a day of celebration and sadness.

Well. Today was it.

Before we talk about today I want to share our experiences of last evening. When we returned home to Savelberg, we sorted through all the art our students had created. In each of our rooms, we made a pile for each student. We ooohh'ed and aah'ed as we looked at their work and thought about the time shared with them in the classroom. I believe Margaret and I were up well past midnight reflecting on all that has occurred over the last two weeks. It feels like we've crammed a semester of learning into a mere ten days and that the kids have all just blossomed.

With that being said, I couldn't do it. I could not pick out a single piece of art from each student in Form 2 to bring back to the States. Margaret was able to do this for Form 1—which is probably a good thing because she had a rowdy bunch. I know both of us had a difficult time sleeping in anticipation of today. It felt so much like coming to the end of something profoundly meaningful.

Margaret, the marathon shopper, did her thing today at Village Market in Muthiaga. Our trusty driver and dear friend, Franco, knew just where to take us. I must admit that I shopped too. I think Margaret and I have started to tire of Nairobi Java as we went there for lunch and it felt lackluster and not nearly as exciting. Both Margaret and I are realizing that we could actually—maybe—eat at other establishments the next time we are here. Maybe.

We arrived at the school with paintings, celebration materials, certificates and pens to hand out to the students as tokens of our gratitude for this experience. The now familiar walk to the school through front yards and raw sewage felt sad as we began to glimpse the end to this chapter of an amazing journey with our students and ourselves. We had gotten used to being accosted by children shouting in their Swahili English, "How are you? How are you?" When we'd respond, a somewhat surprised look would appear on their faces, as if to say, "Oh, they said something?" And then you would hear, "I am good," "fine" or "welcome."

We entered into the flow of the school, feeling like we were a part of it. School never seems to start on time for a myriad of reasons: the children's lunch got served late or the office in which we stored our stuff was locked. I call this "Kenyan time."

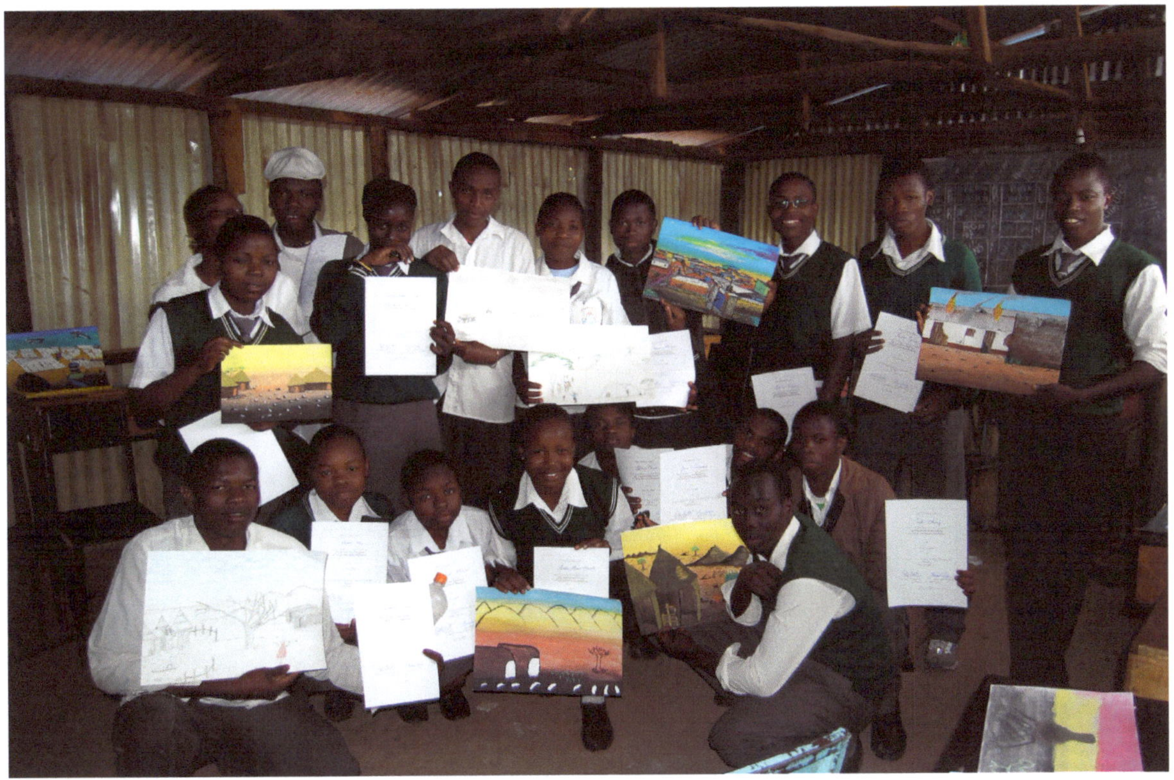

Students share final projects during last day of class.

So, Margaret and I got in the habit of standing at the front door and welcoming each and every one of the students back by shaking hands and saying hello. It was always nice when the students would say hello and grab our hands before we had a chance to greet them. Margaret and I, neither of us having children of our own, now feel like we have two classrooms full of "our kids."

Before the celebration began, Margaret showed her class the pictures she had selected to take home while I gave all the art to my class and asked them to choose what I should take. Each approach worked well given the different temperaments of our classes. My students quietly went through their work, selecting and sharing, and Margaret's class quietly looked at her choices. Then we both introduced them to the "readers" that will reside in the library so they can continue to learn about the art and artists we covered during our time together. Then we both handed out certificates and each student received a pen during a make-shift commencement ceremony. Then, off to celebrate.

Who knew what a big deal three two-liter bottles of soda could be for a group that only usually drinks water. Throw in some chocolates and you've got a big-time celebration on your hands. We talked about the photos they'd taken and we showed them about forty of the thousands of images that they captured. We explained how each photo told a story. They loved it and were so excited; it felt like the school had a bright, shiny light around it.

There was lots of, "I will miss you" and " I learned so much" and "when is the next art class?" When I asked them "What are the three things that I say about you every day?" They immediately responded in loud, clear voices, "I am smart, beautiful and important." Amen to that.

Everyone had talent but some of these students showed exceptional potential. We provided Jacob, the most prolific and advanced artist who we have encouraged to continue, with supplies of his own. He is an amazing artist.

After our celebration, we met with Headmaster Kiambi and Deputy Headmistress Beatrice to debrief on our two weeks. We talked about our curriculum and teaching methods, how we engaged the students and, finally, shared the finished paintings. They laughed at the photos but also recognized the reality of the stories that they told. They were amazed and continued to say how they never knew that their students had such talent.

It was agreed that they would continue to engage these students with art and, with our help, create an art club with time allotted each week for those students who have participated in the Art Immersion program. We have set dates for the second year of the Art in Kibera program to take place in 2009.

I think if you had asked us a week before our first trip to Kenya in 2007 if Margaret and I would be creating an art curriculum and going to teach in the largest slum in Africa, we would have wondered who had spiked your coffee. Now that it has become a reality, (or, as Kiambi said "was a pilot and now is a program that we deliver") I can only share how excited I am to have a future that is connected to these students, all of whom are smart, beautiful and important.

We would like to thank you all for the support, concern, interest and downright love you've given us as it relates to this trip. We carried you all with us in our thoughts. Thank you for keeping us company.

Be well and see you all soon.

Charles and Margaret

ART IN KIBERA

NAIROBI, KENYA 2009

THURSDAY, JULY 16, 2009

Soon we will be in Kenya.

Just a short post to let you know that Margaret and I will soon be leaving to teach art in Kenya. The blogging will begin on July 20th.

We loved your comments last year, please keep them coming.

Much love and appreciation,

Margaret and Charles

TUESDAY, JULY 21, 2009

Karibu nyumbani, global warming and my Kenyan family.

Karibu nyumbani means "Welcome Home" in Kiswahili. It was the first greeting I received upon arriving in Nairobi on Friday night and it feels true; it's just like returning home. I love Kenya. I had such a wonderful feeling walking out of the airport and realizing that I am here again.

Someone asked me, "When will you be collecting Margaret from the airport?" Well, I am happy to say that I collected her last night and am so delighted that we are here to deliver the second year of the Art Immersion program we started together in 2008. Margaret and I continue to be awestruck by the fact that our idea to provide an intensive art education to these "smart, beautiful and important" students at St. Al's is not just a one-time experience but something that is now an ongoing program.

The excitement is building. We've met with Headmaster Kiambi to go over logistics and we went to the Text Book Centre, which is where all schools go to purchase supplies. It is nice to put the money into the Kenyan economy and not have to carry supplies from the US. The people at Text Book Centre are so nice and helpful that it is actually a fun experience. We had our requisite breakfast and afternoon tea at Nairobi Java, so I am feeling fully grounded back in *Our Kenya*.

Let me back up. I arrived Friday evening and went to visit my Kenyan family in Nyeri which is located in Kenya's Central Province. On the way there it became obvious to me that global warming is having a really negative effect on this part of the country, all the way from Nairobi to Nyeri. From Nairobi to Sagana, right outside Nyeri, everything was brown with entire corn crops dead on their stalks. It was hard to see this. Nairobi is normally green at this time of year. My friend, Wangari (some of you know her as Anne) said that this is the worst it has ever been. Awa Ndirangu, Wangari's dad, is a 70-year old agriculturist and he's

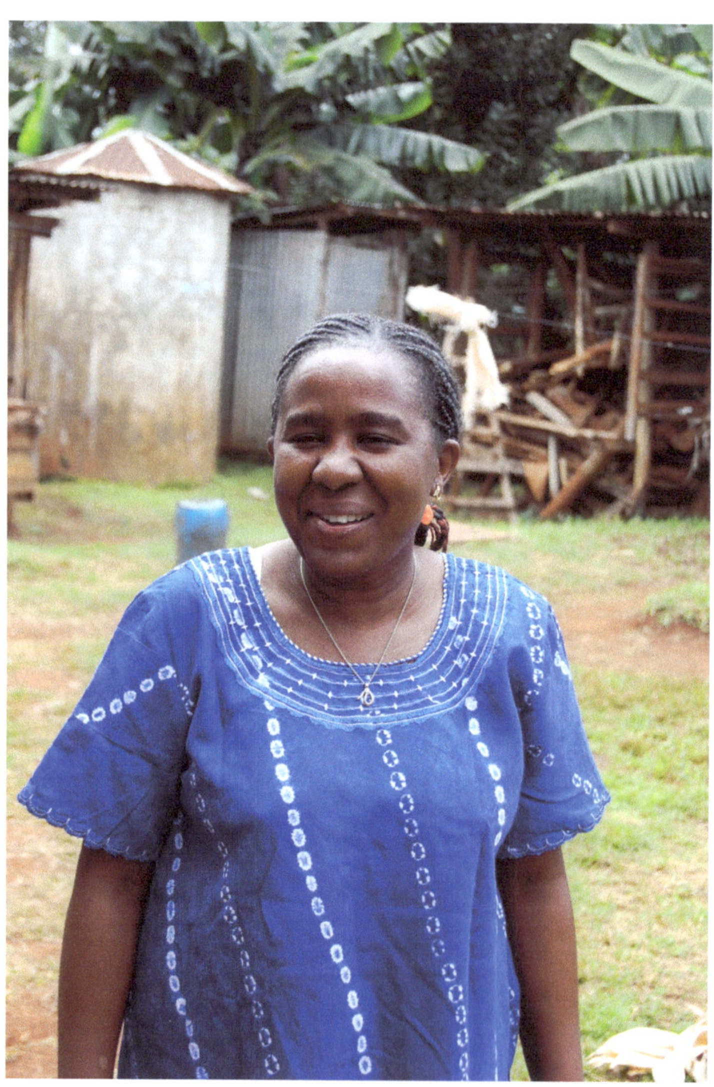

Anne Wangari Ndirangu.

worried. Awa said that this is basically the first year that they don't have corn at this time of year and that the crops are not producing as they normally do. The coffee should be flowering and there should be rain. It is very scary for Kenyans; and as a global citizen, pretty concerning to me, even though in Washington DC, the weather has been abnormally nice. Another side effect of global warming.

The trip to Nyeri was special. I was invited for a Mass being held by the family priest to officially welcome me into my Kenyan family, the Ndirangu's. It is such an honor that a Kenyan family, of whom I have become so fond, wanted to hold a Mass to welcome me into their family. Many of you know that I have a fantastic and wonderful family in the US. Now, to have another family in Kenya - I am filled with gratitude. My first official Kenyan family duty will be to take part in Mr. and Mrs. Ndirangu's 50th wedding anniversary celebration on January 2, 2010. What an amazing gift and honor. Awa (aka, Dad) Ndirangu said he never knew that he would have 7 children, he thought 6 was enough. Most of the family came from all over Kenya for the Mass; those that couldn't be there either sent their spouses or called with best wishes.

To conclude, I am feeling full of life. Having Margaret here to teach with me; being connected to the Ndirangu's; having my first family, the DeSantis's, coming to Nairobi; teaching art to smart, beautiful and important people—wow. We are fortunate.

Charles and Margaret

WEDNESDAY, JULY 22, 2009
The first day of our second year. WOW.

The first day of classes started off without a hitch. Both Margaret and I are overwhelmed, touched, sparked, excited, and proud to be doing something we believe in so passionately.

This year we are actually doubling our teaching time in order to get more time with the students. Last year we taught Forms 1 and 2. Now we are teaching Forms 2 and 3 (last year's students) in addition to the new students in Form 1. Since Margaret had the "freshmen" last year, I get them this year. Hey, it's only fair.

The students continue to exceed our expectations in everything they do. Our day started with warm and excited greetings from the students. The Form 1 class

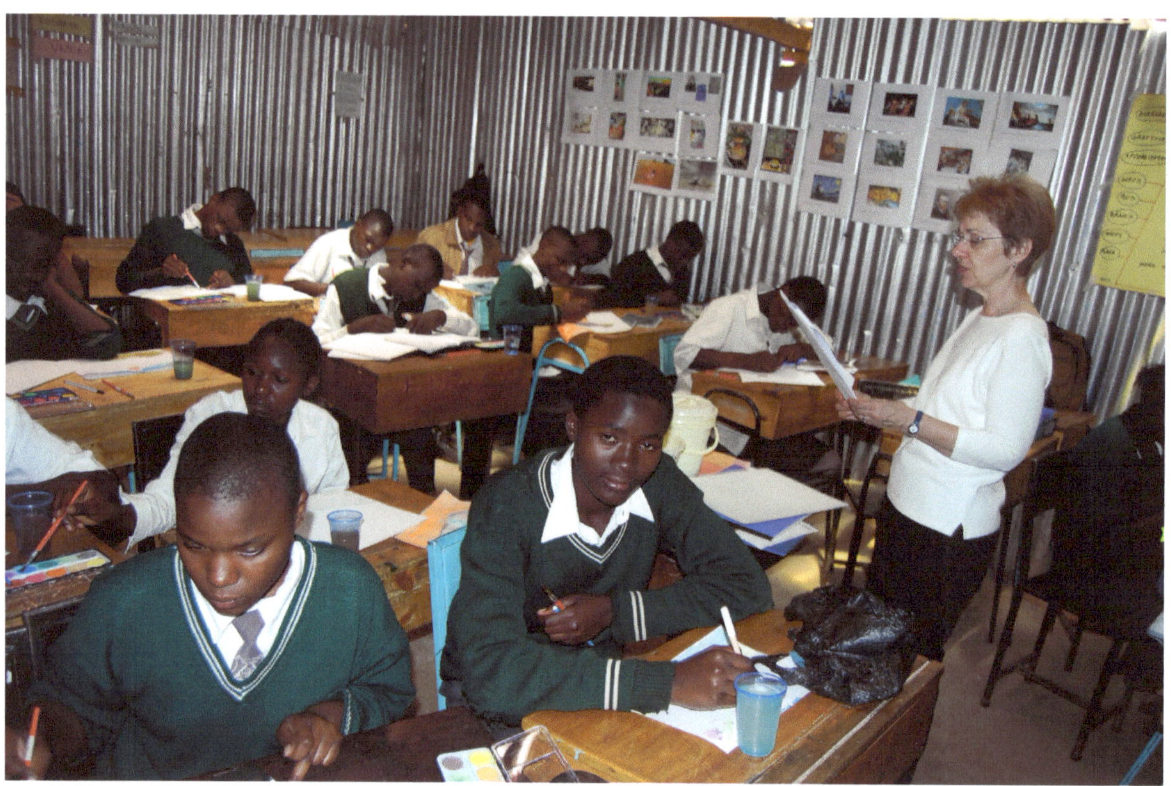

Margaret is back in the classroom at St. Al's for year two of the Art Immersion program.

was excited and very quiet. Margaret's experience with last year's Form 1 group was that they were loud, gregarious and bursting with energy. This class seems subdued. I am sure that this could change as they become more comfortable. I'll be ready for anything. Today, they were excited to engage and when asked what they think "Art" is, they gave canned answers that I know will change as they learn more about what it means to them.

Margaret's Form 2 class has matured since last year. They applauded her when she walked into the class. She was so excited that they remembered the artists we taught them about last year and that they were engaged and ready for more. We could not be happier.

Form 3 was finishing exams today so they will start with me tomorrow after lunch. I cannot wait. This group was wonderful to work with last year and seem really excited to start again. Students from this group—Jacob, Collins and

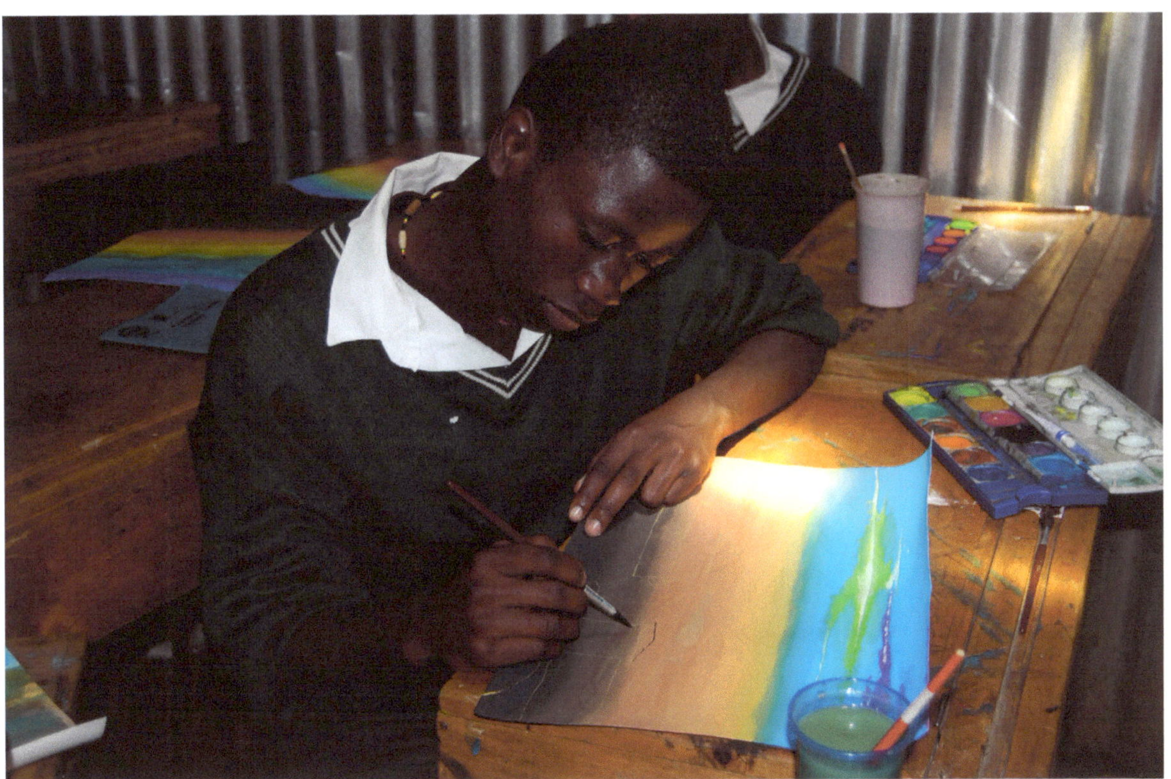

Most students are exposed to watercolors for the first time during their Art Immersion experience.

Hellen—sought us out after class to say that they wanted to update us on their progress. They get together after school on a regular basis and create art. I could not believe that they continued with such ardent enthusiasm; I was nearly in tears. I just stood there, dumbstruck. When I finally pulled myself together, I told them how I was so proud of them and they replied, "No, we are proud of you and Margaret." At that point I think I stopped breathing as I became overwhelmed by that familiar sensation of giving so little to get so much back from these amazing students.

The art that they have created since last year shows definite refinement. It may be a cliché, but it's true: Practice makes perfect. They've had some of their work framed, even sold some of their pictures at a St. Al's event where half the money raised goes to the school and half goes into an account that supports their artistic pursuits.

Margaret and I are so excited to be a part of the process that is creating who they are becoming. I looked at Margaret today and said,"Think about it. We can be with them on this whole journey." She looked at me and said,"Thanks, I guess you made me realize I may do this for a very long time…"

After class we went to lunch with David Dinda. We are in regular contact and it is great to have him so intertwined in my life. He'll be graduating from Social Work College in October and is deciding where he'd like to go to University. He has started the Foundation of Hope to help youth in Kibera give back to their community. He also runs the sports program at St. Al's. Although he may have graduated from St. Al's, he never really left. He's a key part of why they are so successful. He lives his life totally from the perspective that the glass is more than half full. We were talking about success at lunch and he put it simply: "People serve others and experience success when they do what they are passionate about." Enough said!

Starting tomorrow – with the addition of the Form 3 class - we will be teaching as many as 105 students a day. It's hard but certainly one of the most rewarding experiences either of us has had.

Passionately,

Charles and Margaret

THURSDAY, JULY 23, 2009

Day 2: Margaret was running late.

Yes, Margaret was running late but we still made it all happen without a hitch. Two things are particularly great about being here a second time: 1) they expect us, and 2) we know what we're doing. That's an amazing combination. Today we had more time with each of our classes and noticed that they each have a different flavor. Form 1 still seems compliant and excited. We reviewed some history and completed our first project, one that I call Unique Identifier. Students create name plates that represent them as unique humans, just like art and its unique style. They get it. They understand that even when individuals are given the same assignment, how it is interpreted and executed is unique to each person.

Form 2, who offered such challenges last year, is all grown up. They are into art in a way that's both pleasing and exciting to Margaret. They're really pushing to develop their drawing skills. It's rewarding to recognize the foundation that was created last year and to see their readiness and desire to continue toward the next level. Today Margaret shared new skill concepts with them: shading, form and direction of light. They are engrossed.

Form 3 is a smaller but really advanced group. Being experienced students, they were the most mature of our classes last year. Seeing them today, the significance of the self-selection process became evident to me. Out of the 34 students in the class last year, 14 elected to continue with the program this year (for Margaret's Form 2's, 25 of 35 from the prior year are returning). These 14 students immediately started an Art Club after we left last year and have continued to practice and develop their skills. This group has some of the most talented artists. Because of their maturity level, I feel like they are indeed very serious about making a long-term commitment to their art. We talked about sharing personal stories through art. We've seen some of the general, wide-scope stories of Kibera in their art, but I've asked my group to focus internally and to consider sharing their own personal stories in their work, even if it is painful.

The most rewarding aspect for both Margaret and me is that art has become important to them, all of them. They get to choose whether or not to participate; they're in it for themselves, not because it's a requirement.

They want to be here and we're lucky to be here with them.

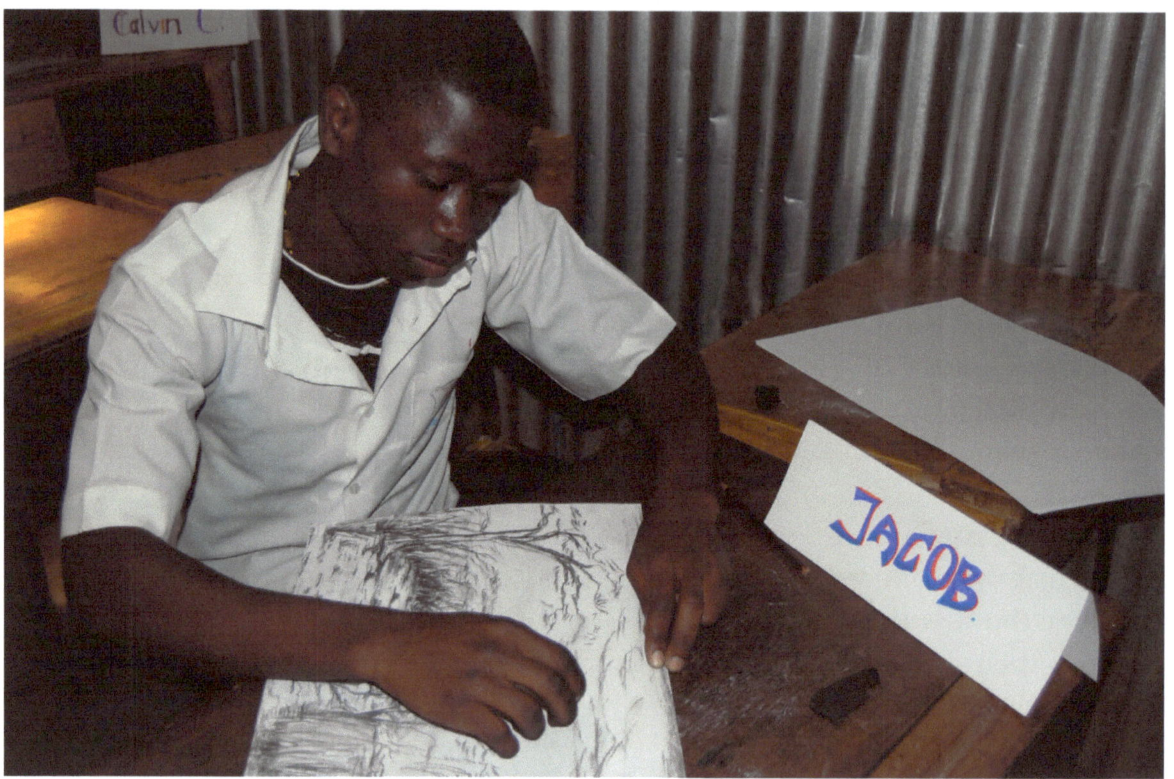

Jacob, a founding member of St. Al's Art Club.

Deputy Headmistress Beatrice continues to state that they had no idea how much talent was here and that it's our program that showed them that this is an important, if not critical, aspect of their students' development. I continue to believe what we learned in 2007, "one person at a time can make a difference."

I think we have quelled our shopping bug. We have identified distinct times that we will go to market to purchase gifts or the Kazuri jewelry we have been asked to purchase. It's really nice to be here and not feel like tourists; on the contrary, to feel a sense of belonging. This is the exact place where we should be.

More to come, hope you are well.

Margaret and Charles

FRIDAY, JULY 24, 2009

Only one week left.

Whoosh. We have completed our first week…I can't believe it. Today was another exceptional day. I'm sure that you are all thinking, "will he get off his soap box already?" But now I understand what educators feel when they see their students transform.

My Form 1 students are so engaged, which is not the experience Margaret had last year. Margaret's Form 2 group is inspired. Today she introduced them to pastels and they loved it. The Form 3 class is so mature, focused and advanced. Today, Hellen, one of the students, handed me a book that tracks attendance for each week of Art club, it begins the week after we left last year. Being an artist myself, I know that making art on a regular basis is critical. They have proved it today.

Our structure this year is 90-minutes of class work followed by 90-minutes of studio work, so they can soak in what they're learning. One of the new mediums that we're introducing is charcoal. When Margaret and I were at the Text Book Centre we couldn't imagine paying four dollars or more for three charcoal pencils. Today, at the start of our studio time with Form 3's, I gave money to Jacob to go to Kibera Road to buy charcoal that has been made on the streets. For 20 Kenyan shillings, he came back with a bag full of Kiberan charcoal and they used it to do their first project. This was amazing.

Tomorrow, Margaret and I are going with David Dinda and about ten of our students to walk through Kibera. We hope to experience a little more than we have before, getting a sense of their lives outside of school. I am really looking forward to it.

This year's experience has made Margaret and I think even more about what's next for this program and, more importantly, what's next in these students' artistic lives. Next year St. Al's will have completed construction of their new school. We're having outstanding results in sub-standard conditions; can you imagine what it will be like to be teaching art in a new school? Over the moon. It was even suggested that the new school might have an ART room. Yes, oh yes, over the moon.

I would also like to share with you that both Margaret and I simultaneously read and finished the book *The Blue Sweater* by Jacqueline Novogratz. She is the Founder of the Acumen Fund which takes a business-centric approach to improving the lives of those in poverty. It has been so appropriate to read this book while here in Kenya. If you haven't read it yet stop reading this blog go out and buy it right now so once you are done with this you can immediately start reading it. It tells a great story, shares a hardy education about working in the third world and answers so many questions. Most importantly, I think, it really demonstrates that it is possible for you to make a difference. At a recent book signing, I had the absolute privilege of meeting the author and talking to her at the dinner that followed. I can't wait to talk to her about the book and our experience here in Kibera.

We spent a charming evening with my friend Wangari which concluded with seeing the new Harry Potter film at Nakumatt Junction for about 6.50 a person. Totally worth seeing, even if you aren't in Nairobi.

Be well and thank you so much for taking this journey with us. It is so nice to be able to share this with you.

Charles and Margaret

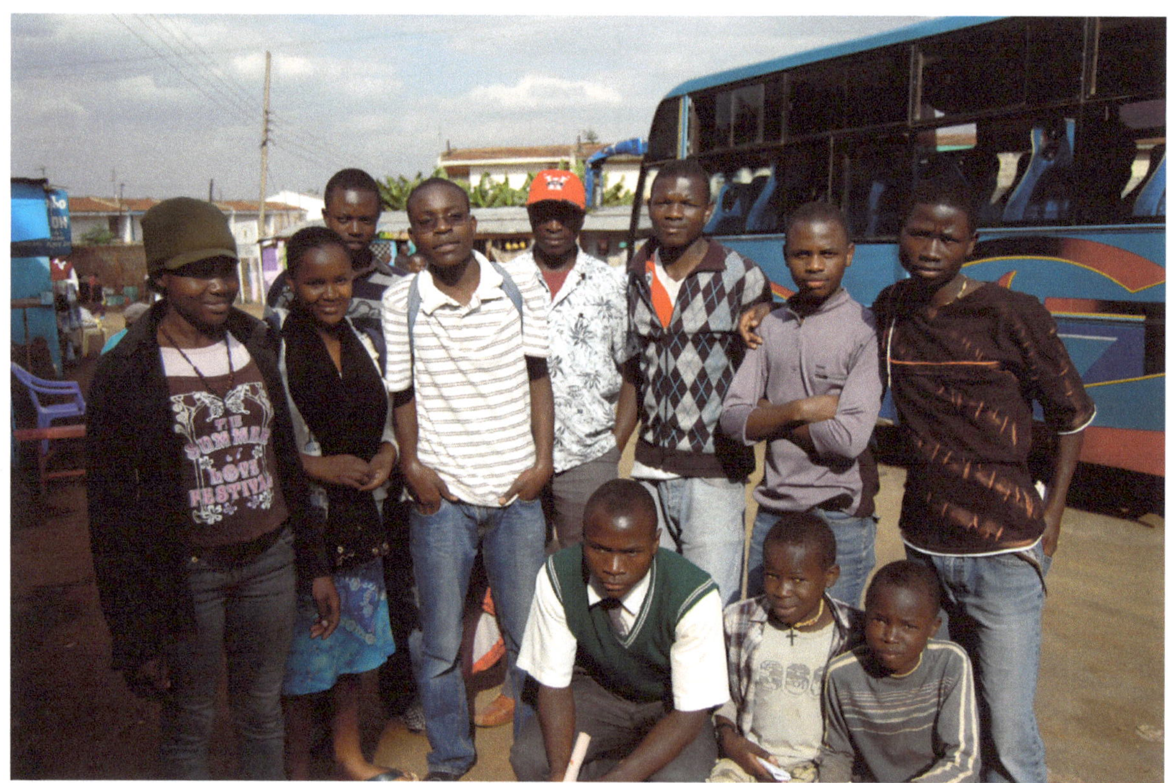

A group of students leads us on a tour of "their Kibera."

MONDAY, JULY 27, 2009
Update through Monday.

This weekend was filled with diverse activities. On Saturday morning we visited Baishara Road downtown where we were able see how Kenyans shop. A good part of the afternoon was spent walking through Kibera with some of our students. They were really excited to share their lives with us. Hellen, David and Jacob walked us through their Kibera and, although we feel really exposed to our students' lives through teaching at St. Al's, we were humbled by how hard their lives are and how they still show up everyday with enthusiasm, hope and readiness.

Saturday night we had dinner with Sr. Mary, Wangari and many of the nuns at Mary Ward Centre where they all live. Sunday was spent at the Masai Market and

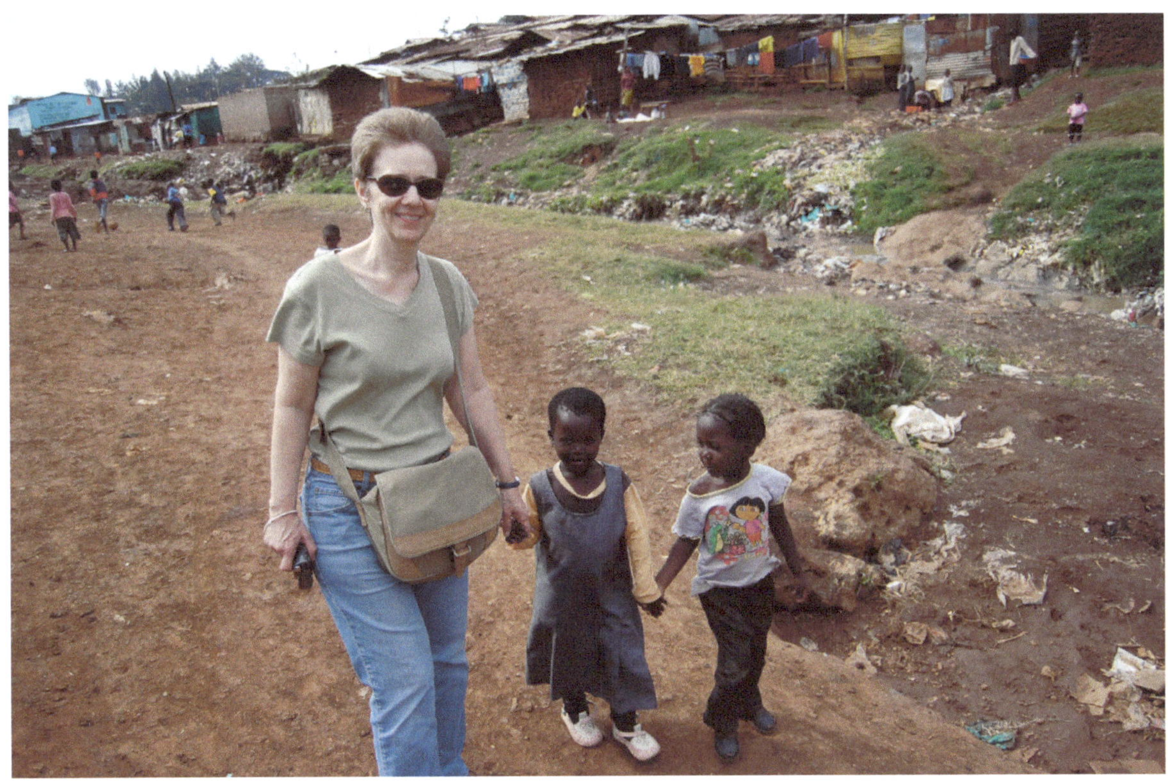

Margaret makes new friends on her insiders' tour of Kibera.

then, thank God, there was rest. It is a lot of work to be here and you need time to process it when time presents itself. I sat and stared at the Ngong Hills and did some painting while Margaret read.

Today is Monday, the beginning of our final week. This is where the rubber meets the road; we have to make sure our curriculum gets covered and all goes according to plan. Today Forms 2 and 3 are using pastels and charcoal; these new mediums are difficult for them. They said that they thought watercolor was hard but that these are far more difficult. The history piece is also much more challenging this year as we're introducing more in-depth information. They get it, they want it, and we are here to provide.

Today we were given the school magazine which mentions Margaret and me as the co-creators of the art immersion program; it characterizes the program as a great success.

Tomorrow, we will have the joy of doing a session with the young kids at the Red Rose School. We teach an art session there each year and, although they don't have art class per se, the teachers do use it in teaching their subjects. The kids there are so fun to teach and spend time with. We will be there in the morning, then a full day of classes at St. Al's and then, if we're still standing, we may take part in the Art Club.

Thanks for taking part in our journey and for reading the blogs.

Be well,

Charles and Margaret

TUESDAY, JULY 28, 2009

A wonderful, frustrating, wonderful day.

So our day started off with teaching the kindergartners at the Red Rose School about portraits. We shared the Mona Lisa with them and they LOVED her. After having received a formal art education, I must admit that I don't get her allure; but all of our students from Kindergarten to Form 3 think she's beautiful. Next, they got to spend time creating portraits of themselves and others. They don't stick within the lines which makes them all the more appealing. They work and laugh and praise everything. I can still hear their sing-song voices ringing in my ears, "Hello to our visitors!" Margaret is a natural with these kids and they are absolutely drawn to her.

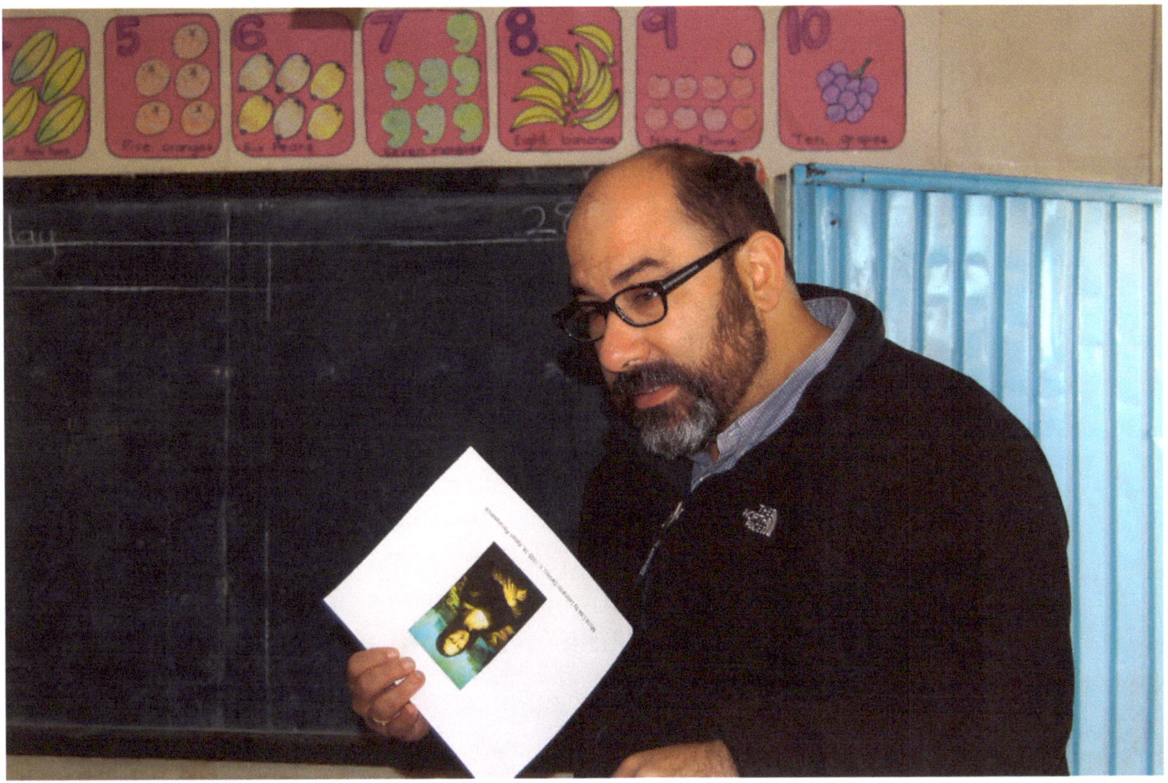

Mona Lisa entrances the students at the Red Rose School.

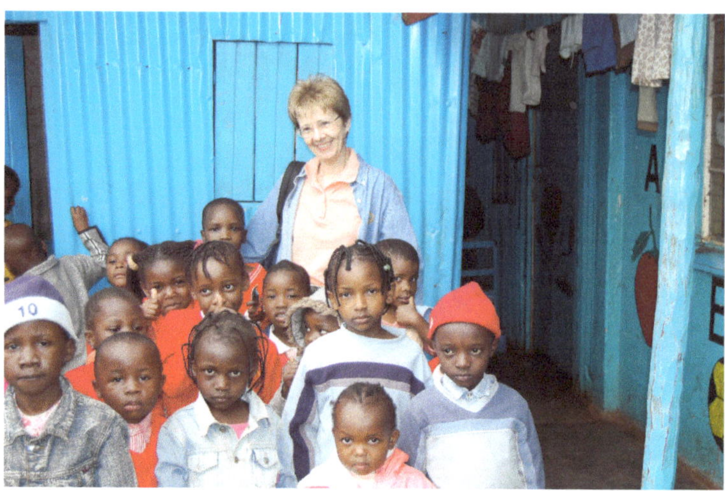

Margaret and her adoring students from the Red Rose School.

At St. Al's we had a scheduling issue come up both yesterday and today. The kids had forum in the church; one day boys, one day girls. The kids who were in church came in late to a class already in progress. So, we ended up needing to stop everything to let them get settled. The desks are placed together so tightly that you have to move them in order to get by. Other students are not in the class but have items locked in the desks that they come to retrieve after church. Some of the students were working on watercolors and found the desk jostling to be highly frustrating with water spilling, etc. It was as frustrating for those of us teaching as it was to those learning. We've been assured that this will not happen during the next few days.

My Form 3 studio session went well. They wanted to continue work after class was over, which they did. They took responsibility for collecting their materials and putting them away. It is also exciting to see Margaret's Form 2 class be so enthusiastic and engaged. The day ended with the Form 3 class being totally focused and Forms 1 and 2 doing well in the studio session. All part of a day's work.

We are basically two days away from concluding this year's program. Friday is our day of celebration and art review. We'll be very busy right up to the finish line. It's obvious that the work we're doing with these students makes an impact. Who knew that we'd be planning Art Immersion 2010 and thinking out even further than that?

More to report later…

Charles and Margaret

WEDNESDAY, JULY 29, 2009

Time is speeding by.

It's Wednesday, another rewarding day filled with hard work. I am sure Margaret is well aware, having taught art eight hours a day for twelve years, but I am just discovering how hard it is to teach daily. And we're only teaching four hours a day. Part of the challenge is this environment and how much work it is just to get set up each day, getting the supplies out, etc. There's also an emotional element that is exhausting although extremely rewarding. Case in point: today a child from the school who lives nearby was on the landing between two flights of stairs crying and crying because he couldn't get down. I went up to the landing, handed him off to Momma Margaret who then carried him home. Minutes later he was back

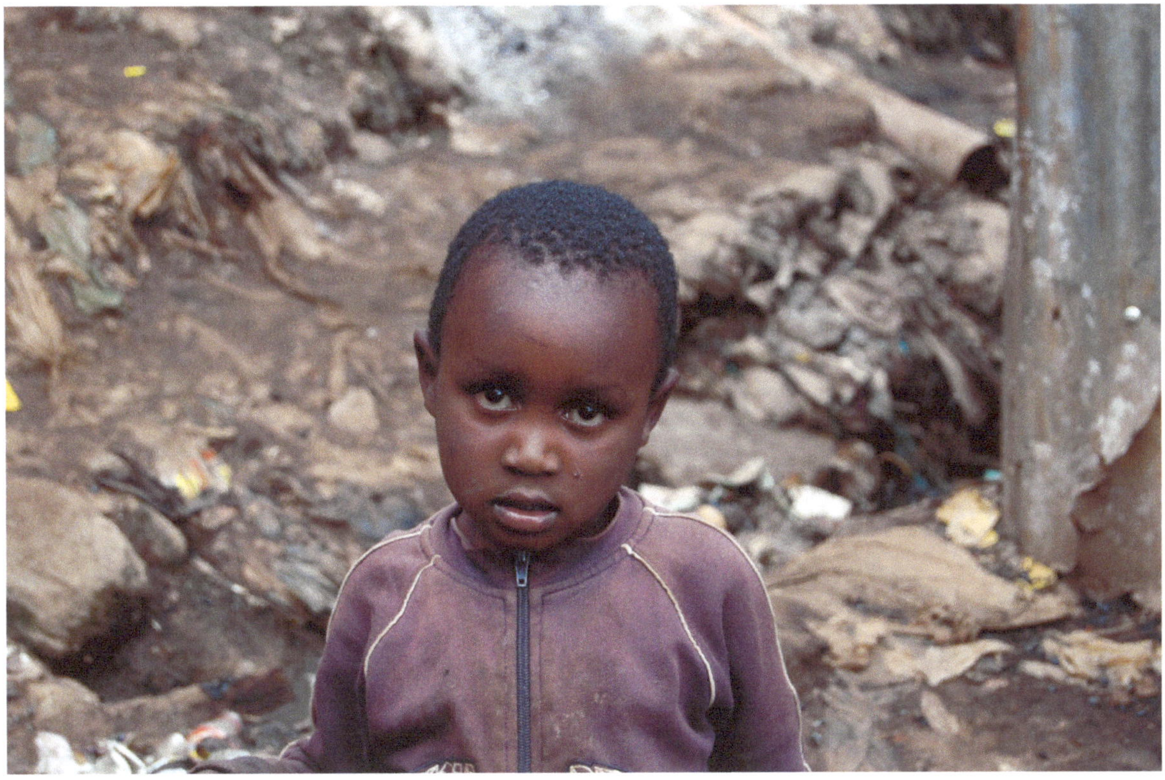

A young resident of the Kibera slum.

in the school sitting on a chair at the doors of our classrooms smiling and waving, asking over and over again, "how are you?, how are you? how are you?" I love this and, at the same time, these are the elements of daily life at this school that so many people will never experience.

Today felt like we were racing to get all the work done. I am realizing that we had eight days this year compared to ten last year. We really need the full ten days, regardless of the fact that we have more total teaching hours this year. We actually need the days to deliver the curriculum; this truncated amount of time leaves us very little room for flexibility. It just makes us push, push, push. I quoted him last year, I'll quote him again next year - Phil Boroughs advised us that it is never going to be as you planned it. That continues to be the best advice we've received, that is, outside of "don't drink the water unless you bought it bottled."

Today all the classes were creating at full tilt. We've had to work very hard to squeeze in our history and technique education in addition to time for practice. The most essential elements that need to be delivered are composition, genre, medium, and an overview of historical periods. But, we're doing it. The advanced students, Forms 2 and 3, are doing final projects on high-grade paper and Form 1 is doing lots of painting on, what we call, practice paper. They are all working so hard with such commitment, taking full advantage of this opportunity while it is here. The final projects are amazing and will certainly be great to bring back to the US to help raise money for the school.

We are learning to speak Kenyan. After class this afternoon, the Art Club asked to meet with Margaret and me. At the start of the meeting we told the group how proud we are of them and that we'll remain committed to their progress. They were thankful to learn that all of the remaining art supplies for this year would be given to them.

Now, back to speaking Kenyan, this is what I am talking about: Hillary was the club's appointed speaker and asked us, "What are your thoughts about the club taking a field trip to see a museum or gallery either while you are here or even when you aren't here?" We responded that we thought this was a fine idea but given that we are leaving this Friday it would be best for them to go on their own. But I knew that this wasn't the real question they were asking. So, I said, "I am not sure I am answering your question, since you are not being direct." Then they clarified somewhat and asked if we would "support" them going. I continued to dig and finally asked, "Do you need money to do this and is that what you are asking for?" They all said yes. Then we talked about how to be direct and to ask for what you need. Helping them have a voice is important. They acknowledged that it is very Kenyan to be indirect and dance around the request. We told them that we are more than glad to support this effort and gave them an assignment: Collin is to figure out how much money they need and Hellen is to focus on where they might go. At dinner, Margaret said, "What if they come back with the idea to go to the MOMA or the Metropolitan Museum of Art in New York?!" We laughed and both of us thought it would be great. Maybe this will be something to look forward to.

The world is a small place. Tonight I met someone at Nairobi Java who was wearing an unusual pair of Kenyan Safari boots - the same boots that I recently bought so I would be unique at home (go figure). I introduced myself and we joked about being fashionable in our respective home towns. He is a Kenyan who lives in Paris and I'm in DC. I gave him my card and said "Send me a picture of you wearing your boots in front of the Eiffel Tower and I'll send you one of me wearing mine in front of the White House." He said he is in Kenya working with a school in Kibera on a photojournalism project. And, lo and behold, the Journalism Club of St. Al's is opening an exhibit tomorrow that he was part of organizing! Small world. Margaret and I are particularly excited about the project because last year we engaged the students with photography and three of the six photojournalists are our students from last year.

Hope all is well.

Charles and Margaret

THURSDAY, JULY 30, 2009

Last day of classes.

Today was hard. You see the commitment, the desire and the progress made in such a short amount of time and you just want to continue. It makes me wonder: what would it be like to have these students engaging in art as part of their curriculum all year round? The Art Club is certainly an important step in that direction. Forms 2 and 3 had final projects to do and, I have to say, they are truly impressive. In fact, some visitors who saw the students' work asked, "Have they had formal training?" To which I responded, "Yes, they started in the introductory art immersion program and now they are in the advanced art immersion program!" We all laughed. These students have very distinct styles. The things that they

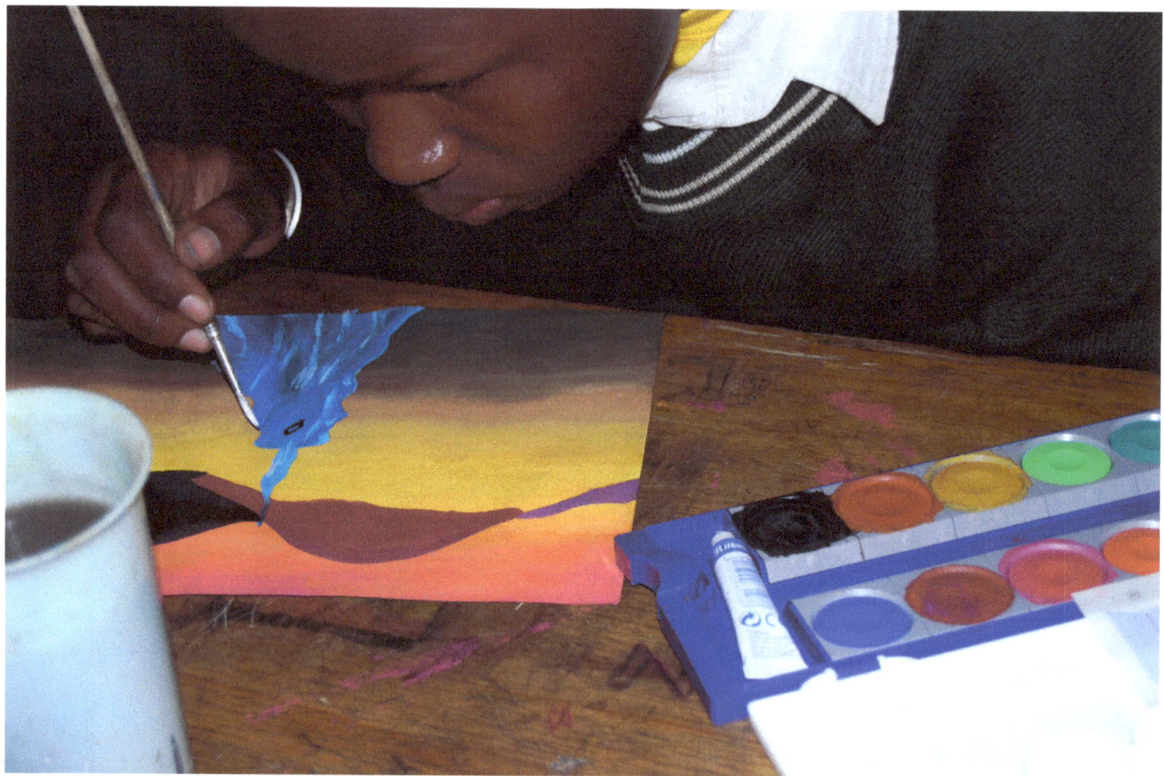

Student engrossed in completion of the final project.

understand, the things they want and the things to which they aspire continue to inspire Margaret and me.

As we walked into the school today, Margaret and I realized that, as long as the new school is built as scheduled, this would be the last time we'd walk into this particular building to teach. We will always carry with us the awkward, dissonant beauty that we have encountered on our daily walk to class - the raw sewage, associated smells, trash, and displaced humanity partnered with the radiance of the people and the hope that exists here.

When we returned from lunch, the students were buzzing about and starting to paint, knowing today was the last class. Tomorrow will be assembly, rewards and art review before they go on a two week break.

Margaret's students continue to be so different than they were last year. She has one artist that is especially prolific. You can't help but stare in amazement at his use of color and distinct style. This is such progress.

My Form 3 class wanted to know what happens next after they graduate from St. Al's. Do they continue to progress? Or, do they just abandon their art education? Two things came to mind for me: 1) we haven't even begun to scratch the surface of art education and 2) hmmmm, maybe the Kibera Art Institute? I love this idea but have to get re-grounded back in the States to see if it's just my adrenaline and blind faith that thinks this is a great idea, or if this a model that could really work. More on this to come.

This evening ended at the Kuona Art Trust where the journalism club had a showing of their projects. The photos where fantastic One of Margaret's students is part of the club and produced really great work.

Paul O'Callaghan (a volunteer), Collin (a professional photographer – and great guy - who's married to a Kenyan) and many others made this event a reality. (Margaret and I talked about an art show as a next step in the program – we'll probably need to add at least another week to make this happen.) The drama club did a marvelous performance of traditional dances. Also during the program, Margaret and I were recognized – humbling and nice, all at once.

I shall write one last entry after our celebration tomorrow and then we will have concluded our second year of the program. Thanks for being on this journey with us.

Be well,

Charles and Margaret

FRIDAY, JULY 31, 2009
Our last day at St. Al's in Kibera.

Today we walked down the path from Kibera Road to St. Al's for the last time this year - probably forever. If all goes as planned, next year we'll be teaching in the new school. Without a doubt, the last day is always hard. The students are so smart, willing and able that you want to take them home with you. It's hard not to think about who they are, what they've gone through and all that they've accomplished.

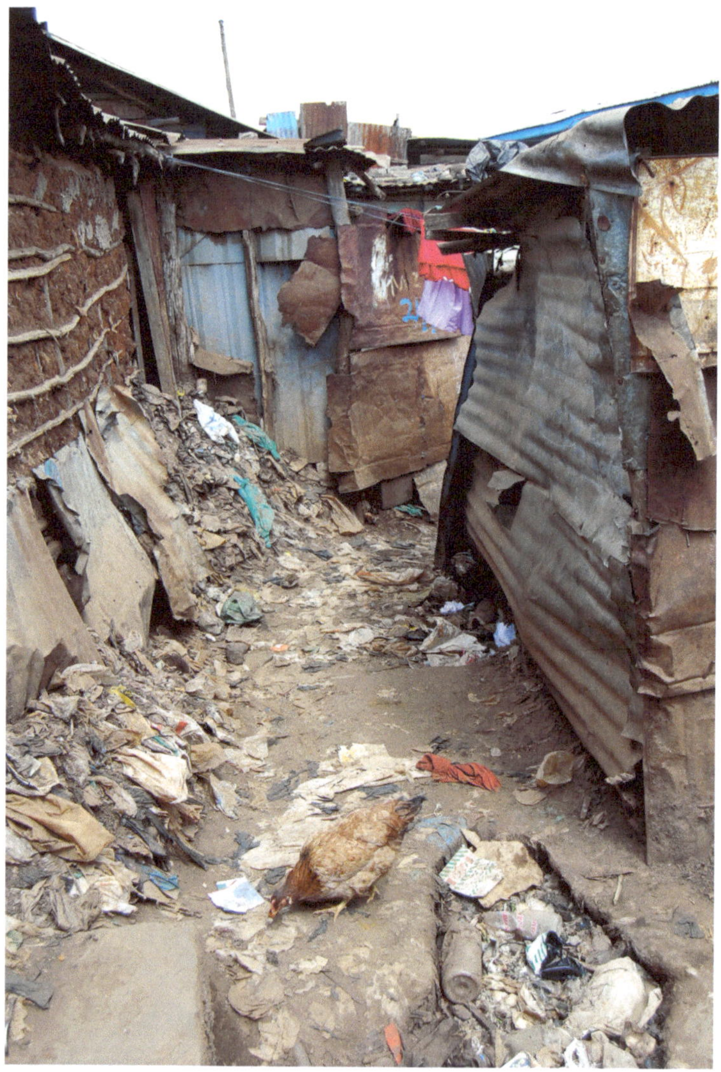

The pathway to St. Al's.

As is now our tradition, the last day of class is focused on art review and celebration. Form 1 rearranged the room so we could spread their art out so everyone could look at it. We gave out certificates to each one of the students. They really love this proof of their accomplishment. There was one student who started late so I didn't have him on my list as I was creating the certificates. Thank God we had made extra copies for just such cases. Then after we reviewed the art and distributed the certificates, we had a grand celebration that consisted of ginger snaps, chocolate and soda. This seemed to be a winning combination as it was greeted with much excitement and applause.

In Form 2, Margaret reviewed their work and handed out certificates as well, then, her class sang songs to her. It was really wonderful. It is plain to see that these students love Ms. Margaret. Jill, one of the senior faculty, came by to wish us well and thank us. She loves this program and has a personal passion for art; she knows all the artists that we teach. She actually went to a school in Kenya that

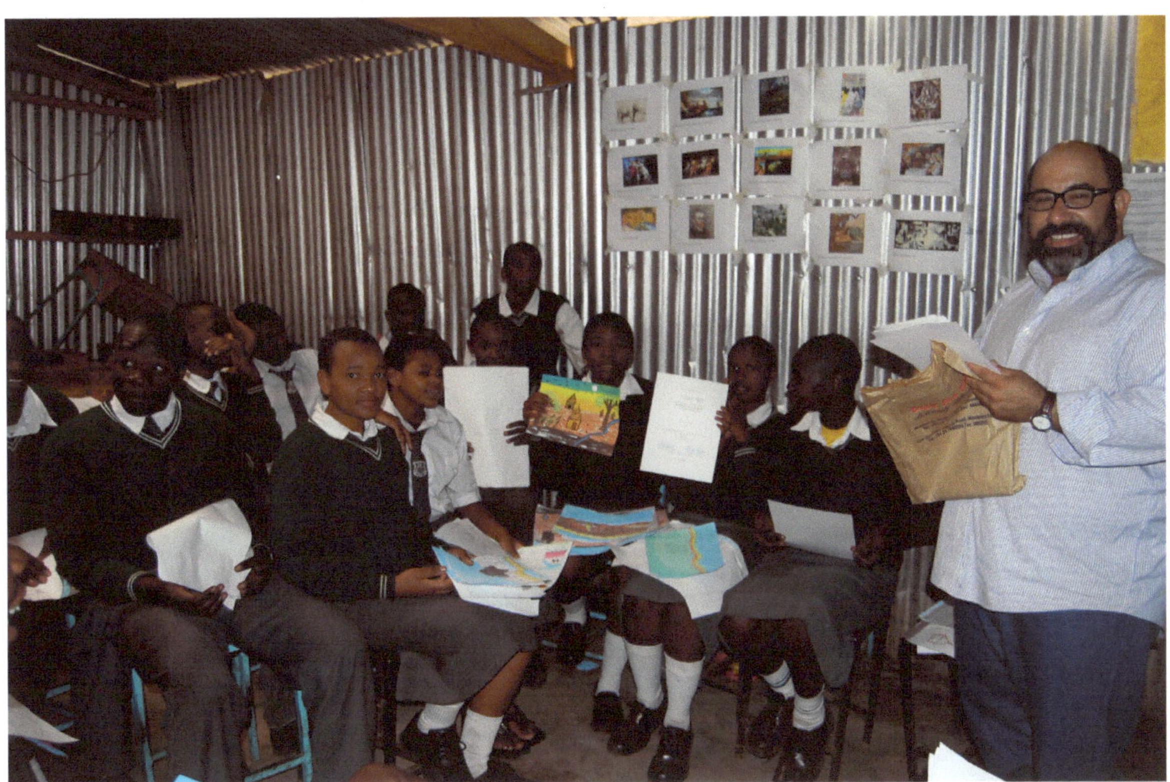

Our students proudly celebrate their accomplishments and share their final projects.

had a special program. If it had not been for her request for us to bring art to St. Al's, this program would have never been started.

Form 3 had a larger classroom with fewer students, so they were able to spread the art all around the room. We went through and talked about the differences and how they had each developed as artists. It is funny to see them as a talkative and quirky bunch. Having been in the art and drama clubs in high school (no surprise, right?) they seem familiar to me.

Today I asked the Forms 1 and 3 what they should always, without fail, remember from our class: They are Smart, Beautiful and Important. They know that this applies to their art as well; what they create is smart, beautiful and important, too. One student shared that she also learned that art is "beautiful, storytelling and artistic." You get to take from it what you want. That is the beauty of sharing and teaching.

After class, Jacob, one of our students in Form 3, wanted to share his home and family with us. It was incredibly moving. When they invite you in, it is such an honor. Having lost his parents, Jacob's aunt has taken him and his siblings in. We were welcomed so graciously into their home, with little means and so many needs they offered food and asked if they could get us anything. The hospitality is overwhelming to me and in stark contrast to the harsh realities they inhabit. A reminder of how fortunate we are and how challenging life is for them.

As we were leaving the school today - after the visit with Jacob's family - we walked up the path back to Kibera Road in silence. We were already beginning to miss it. The filth and the smells, the children with bare feet walking through raw sewage, the products being sold on the street, the sing-song sounds of the children saying "how are you?" over and over again. The beauty of the students, their hope and ambition, the delightful faces of the people that we've met and the new family that we have formed.

David Dinda came to say good-bye and it was hard. David was also very excited because the soccer team he coaches won their match last night. It was on the news and in The Nation (a Kenyan newspaper) today! I am so proud of my Kenyan son.

We are now at Pedro Arrupe preparing for our departure this evening. We will join the Jesuits at Hekima College before we leave to celebrate the Feast of St. Ignatius, watch the change of guard to the new Father Superior of the Jesuits of East Africa and say good-bye to some friends. I could not imagine a better way to end this day or this journey.

As we conclude our second year, we realize how fortunate we are to do this work. It is not only important and meaningful, it is also a privilege to serve these smart, beautiful and important Kenyans. In our service to the students of St. Aloysius of Gonzaga, we receive more than we could imagine in return. This is true reciprocity.

We have been fortunate to have this experience and look forward to what 2010 will bring us when we return. More to come…

Be well,

Charles and Margaret

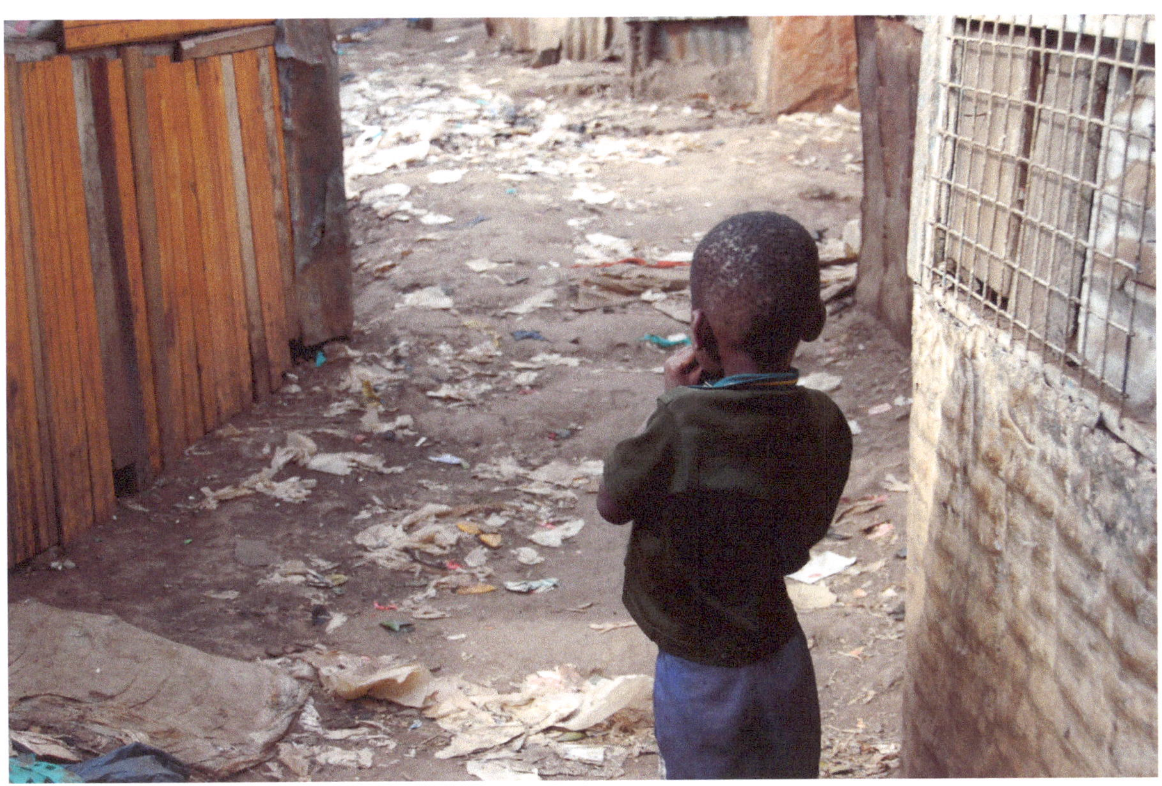

ART IN KIBERA

NAIROBI, KENYA 2010

MONDAY, JUNE 14, 2010

We leave in less than 48 hours.

We'll soon be on our way to teach art at St. Al's for the third consecutive year. We are excited to be on our way and find that this year, as with each other year, everything seems to be falling into place. Flawlessly!

I subscribe to the belief system of "ask and you shall receive." This year, not only have we received more money than we have over the past two years, but we've also had some unique giving occur.

About eight months ago I met Count Von Faber-Castell who is CEO of the venerable Faber-Castell company of Germany that produces almost all #2 pencils used in schools. The more mature among us may recall having used their products in the classroom and those of us that are artistically-inclined definitely know Faber-Castell for producing some of the finest art supplies available. Well, when I met Tony (aka, The Count) he said if there was anything we needed for the program to simply let him know. As you can imagine, I took him up on his offer and emailed him a week and half ago asking for charcoal pencils. He promptly replied instructing me to provide his office in Germany with a list. At this point, I contacted Margaret who formulated the list that I then blindly sent on. Shortly thereafter Margaret asked me, "Which items from the list did you ask for?" I gulped and said, " I thought you wanted all of it." Ooops. She thought I would select only a few things. Next thing you know, Tony's assistant emails saying that she hopes I receive the supplies before we depart. They arrived today: some of the finest and most beautiful supplies available in the marketplace. I cannot wait to share these incredible tools of the trade with our students!

This spring I participated in a residency program called Insight Onsite at Frank Lloyd Wright's famous architectural masterpiece, Fallingwater. While there I befriended the Vice President and Curator for the property, Lynda and Justin. While having lunch with them today, I shared that Margaret has placed Frank Lloyd Wright on our third year curriculum. They were so excited that they are sending post cards displaying examples of Wright's work and a powerpoint presentation to share with the students.

I cannot begin to express my gratitude for the generous support of the work that Margaret and I so love to do. It is an honor for us to deliver art education to

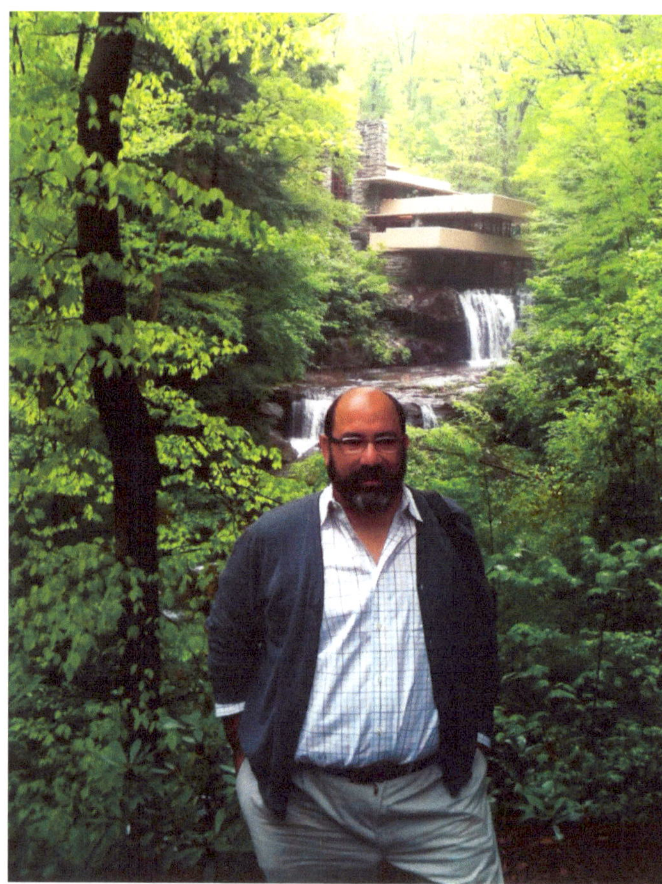

Charles DeSantis at Fallingwater in Pennsylvania, Spring 2010.

the smart, beautiful and important students of St. Al's and the kids of the Red Rose School.

The next time you'll be getting a post from us we'll be on the ground in Kenya preparing to start class in the new school. Can you believe it? I am so excited and a little sad. I love walking through Kibera to our old school; seeing all the familiar faces of the residents of the area in which we teach. I will want to go visit them and say hello. However, I am beyond excited that the students now have wonderful accommodations in which to receive their education. They deserve this and so much more.

With gratitude for all your love and support as we begin the third year of our journey.

Charles and Margaret

SATURDAY, JUNE 19, 2010

It's so great to be back.

It has been wonderful to be back in a place that owns a piece of both Margaret's and my heart. As far as travel was concerned, it was a fairly uneventful journey. The one thing I did realize, from sitting directly behind Margaret, was that when she doesn't sleep well she moves about a great deal. This is just an observation, not a complaint. On the second leg from Amsterdam to Kenya, we were able to sit next to each other. Economy KLM was just great and, as promised, Margaret did not fall asleep and drool on me. It frequently happens with people I don't even know on airplanes, so it really wouldn't have been a problem.

We arrived in Kenya and, as always, Margaret was ultra prepared. She had her visa from the Kenyan Embassy in DC and I, of course, did not. When, during my

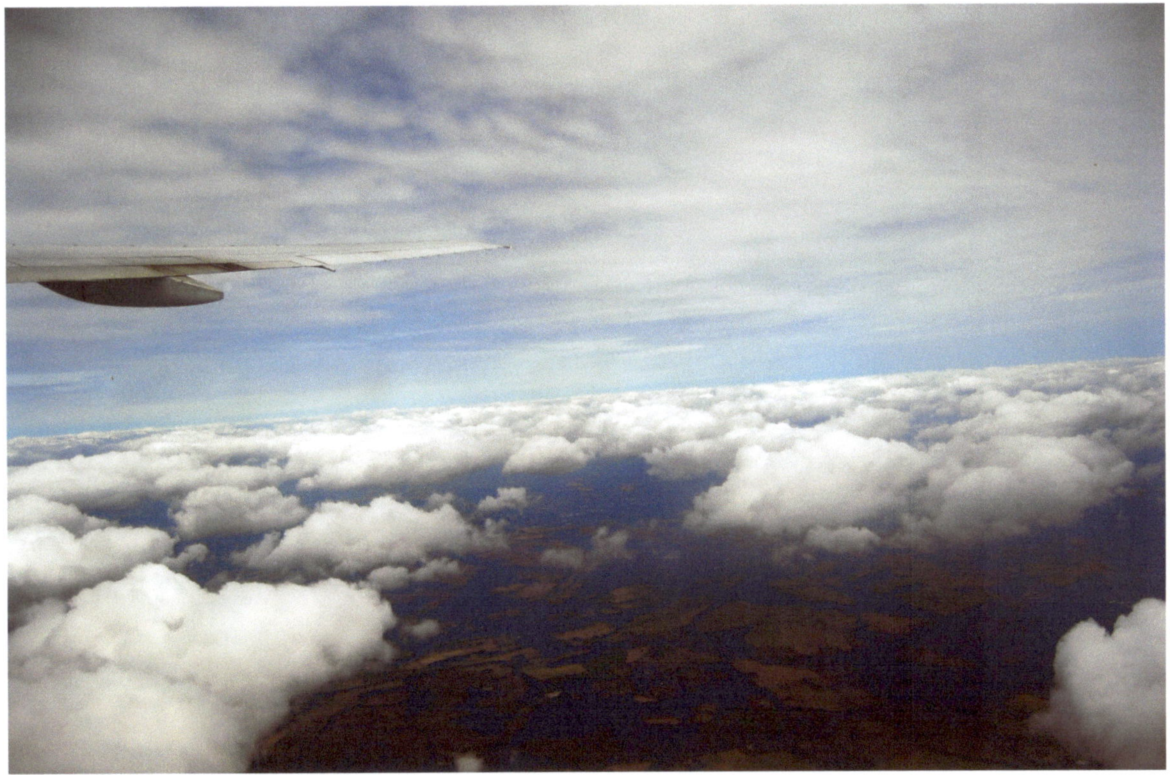

En route to Kenya, June 2010.

last trip in December, I realized how easy it was to get one on the spot, that piece of planning went right out of my head. Why go get two pictures, a money order, fill out a form, wait in line, and have to return in eight days to pick it up when you can show up with $25 USD and smile for the camera? After sixteen hours on a plane, what's another hour? If this isn't a perfect example of why it takes all types of personalities to get things done, I don't know what is. As it relates to this Art in Kibera program, Margaret is the Yin to my Yang. We are a perfect complement. As I continue to see this program grow, succeed and serve, I realize it is because of our unique approaches and the different things that we own in making this happen. It takes all types; I definitely see this with Margaret and me.

Per established protocol, we were met at the airport by our dear friend and chief transportation officer, Franco Sego, who was graciously and happily waiting for us to arrive. All I can say is that when I see Franco's face upon coming out of the terminal, all is right with the world. He has such a wonderful demeanor and feels like a stalwart representative of Kenya to us.

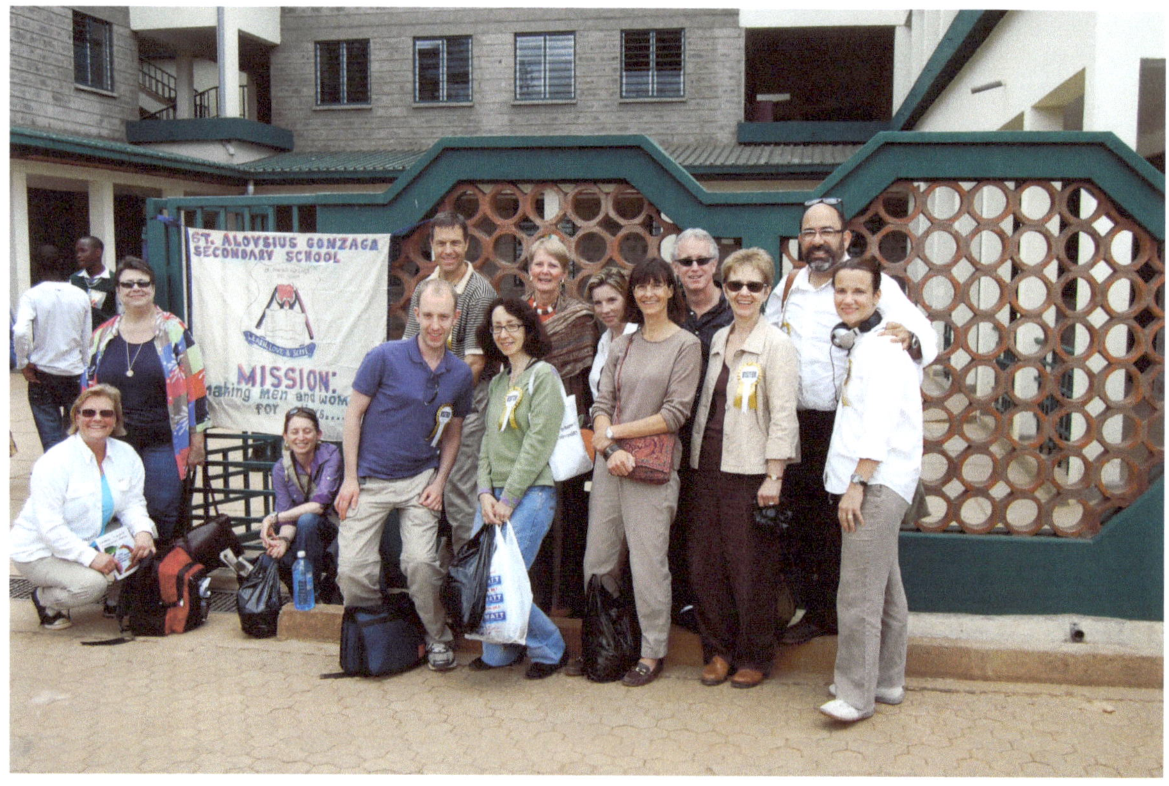

Georgetown University's 2010 Kenya Immersion Group outside of St. Al's.

We were carefully delivered to Pedro Arrupe Jesuit Home where we are fortunate to (temporarily) reside amongst the beautiful Jesuits, Ngong Hills, lovely grounds and the most amazing people. We also are surrounded by nature, which is to say that there are dogs serenading us at this very moment. You should hear them. They are howling like they're in a chorus; it is something we've come to expect each night. There are three beautiful, friendly tan dogs on the grounds that like to accompany you wherever you may be going. Then there are the guard dogs that are behind a gate but definitely let you hear it at night when they sense a threat.

Friday morning we were able to see Georgetown's 2010 Kenyan Immersion Group that is staying here on the same property at the Mwamgaza Retreat Center. We went up to see them after we had breakfast and were invited to join the group for lunch and to meet and talk with Stanley Gazemba, who is a Kenyan writer recently recognized on NPR. Gazemba has written many books with one coming out soon in a republished format. It was intriguing. Next we headed to the Nakumatt which is only – and I am not exaggerating - the greatest store on earth. Dare I call it the Walmart of Kenya? I don't think I'm too far off. We bought all the requisite things one needs: water, wine and new cameras (Margaret's died). We then headed off to Pedro Arrupe for dinner and took part in the nightly reflection with the 2010 immersion group. After having visited Kenya originally in this format it's interesting to see the dynamics of another group. They are a wonderful set of people, most of whom I know from Georgetown and a few that I am meeting for the first time. One of the participants made our evening when she said, "It is nice to have you here and important that you take part." Feeling welcome is always nice but it's especially meaningful when it's by a community you're connected to.

Today, Saturday, has been an interesting day. On our original trip in 2007, Margaret was sick when our group went to see the Kweto Home for Boys but today she was able to join the 2010 group on their visit. As you'll recall, the Kweto home is for boys from the surrounding slums who are overcoming a drug or glue-sniffing addiction; a safe haven for them while they get it back together. It was one of the hardest elements of the trip for me in 2007 and Margaret experienced it today. The boys just want love - it is so clear. I am glad that Margaret got to experience this.

My mid-morning was spent in a more superficial non-Kenyan centric pursuit: searching for a tailor to make me a suit. Franco knows everyone and, of course, has a cousin who is a tailor. I'll need a suit on my return trip as I'm attending the Caine Prize for African Writing at Oxford on July 5. And…I didn't bring a suit. Details, details (details that Margaret would have remembered!). Franco took me to a tailor and after that we joined the 2010 group for lunch as we fetched Margaret. I was also delighted to able to see Sarah and Jamie, graduate students in Conflict Resolution from Georgetown's Government Department. They will be here for seven weeks interning and making connections. Jamie worked with me on GAIN (Georgetown African Interest Network)which is a collaborative program consisting of all Georgetown entities, people and departments, engaged in Africa-centric work both professionally and personally. I am the Co-convener of this program along with Scott Taylor, Professor in African Studies. It was great to see these two Hoyas and I am sure we will see them often.

After this, we were off to purchase art supplies at the Text Book Centre for the third year in a row. In alignment with my "ask and thou shall receive" theme, it had never before dawned on me to ask for a teaching discount! Well, viola. One of the heads of the store came over and said, "Of course!" and we left the store swimming in gratitude.

Then my suit pursuit continued. I was thrilled to find a beautiful suit at Sir Henry's Menswear, the oldest clothier for men in East Africa. They were offering a 140 super count wool Italian suit, with three shirts and three ties for $217 USD. I was in shock. It fit very well and I knew it was meant to be. I am now ready for Oxford and no longer worried. Time flies by while you're here and I envisioned myself getting to London with very little time to get properly outfitted for this event.

Next, Margaret and I had tea at Nairobi Java and meandered around, came home and rested before having dinner with the group. It's great to be staying at the same place where we were originally introduced to Kenya. We've stayed here three of the four times we've been here and feel very much a part of this community. It's also great to have 14 other people from Georgetown here and to know that you have a place in the world that wants you to be in it as much as you want to be there.

Margaret and I are unprepared for what tomorrow will bring. It's the grand opening of the new school. Those of you that have followed the blog in past years know that we taught in a shanty-style school with corrugated roofs, dirt floors, little to no electricity and the most amazing students ever. With all its "third world charm," we loved the school. The new school is one that we've heard is nothing short of amazing; one that people in the States would love to be taught in. What a well-deserved gift for the students. There are so many who have been essential to making this happen, a few who come immediately to mind are Martha and Dave Swanson and Phil Boroughs, SJ . Hats off to these individuals and to all who have contributed to the well-being and development of this school. The grand opening coincides with the feast of St. Aloysius of Gonzaga,which is the name "saint" of this school. I am sure it will be an emotion-filled celebration.

We start school on Monday, the third year of Art in Kibera and I cannot wait to share this experience with the Smart, Beautiful and Important students of St. Al's. The connection we've come to have with them is remarkable and worth all the money in the world.

Thanks for being here with us.

Charles and Margaret

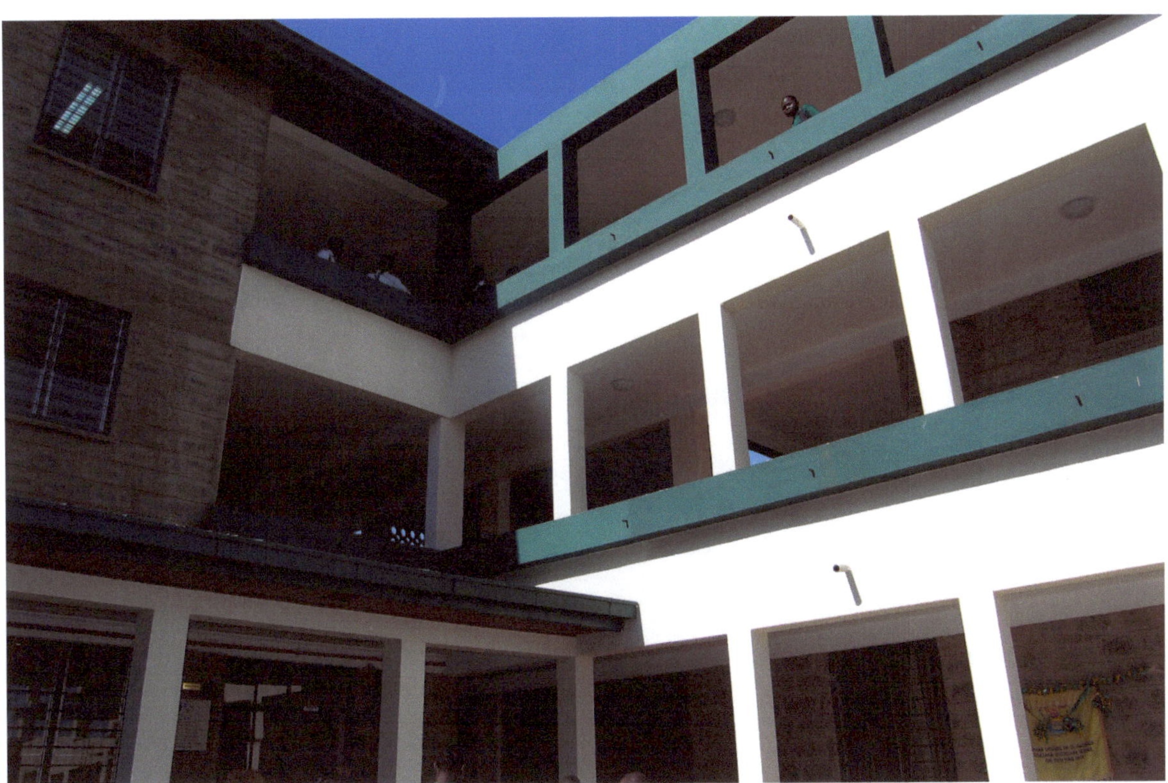

The new school.

SUNDAY, JUNE 20, 2010

The new school

What an amazing experience. We arrived at the school at 10am this morning. I knew exactly where we were going but when we turned the corner, I thought, "Hmmm, they must have built a three story apartment building near the new school," since I remembered only a two-story plan for the new school. Nonetheless, we parked the car and walked inside. I was speechless, absolutely speechless. As we entered the building, three of my students came running up to Margaret and me. "You are here and you must see that we have an art room. Charles and Margaret, we have an art room!" The students were so proud of their school- I was so proud of their school - and the celebration that ensued was joyous and heartfelt.

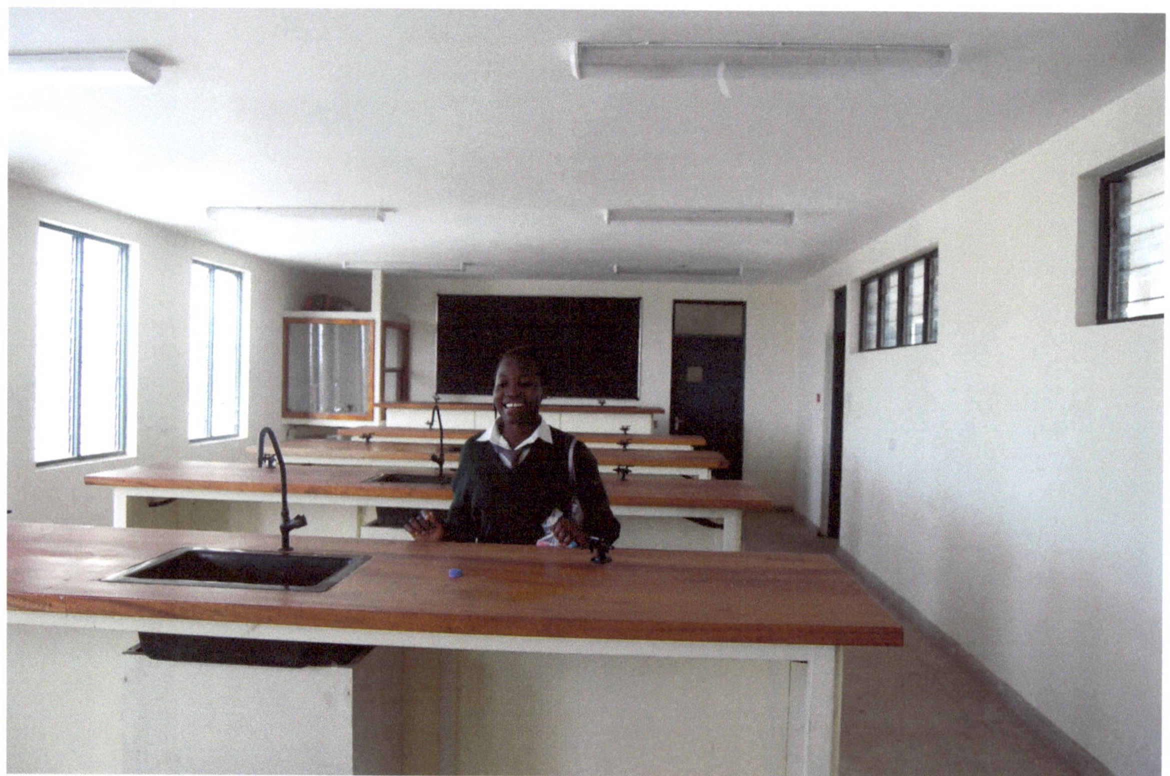

A student enjoys one of the many classrooms in her new school.

I was so wrapped up in everything that was going on, I just walked about hugging our students, shaking hands with new students, meeting guardians, parents, Jesuits (both local and from afar), benefactors from Wisconsin and Chicago, Friends of St. Al's and on and on. When we walked into the art room, Hellen, one of the Form 4 students screamed our names, hugged us and said, "You are here, you are here." This happened time and again throughout the day. In writing this, it's the first time I've had time to myself to process today's events and it has finally hit me; there are tears streaming down my face. This school has the most amazing resources that one could imagine and I don't have to add "amazing for Africa" to this statement. It is wondrous. Any American student would be proud to be educated in this beautiful school. The layout is welcoming, the feeling is warm and the heart of the school is ever-present. There is a chapel in the middle of the school and it beats strong as the heart of this institution. They have a real school. It's shocking and fantastic.

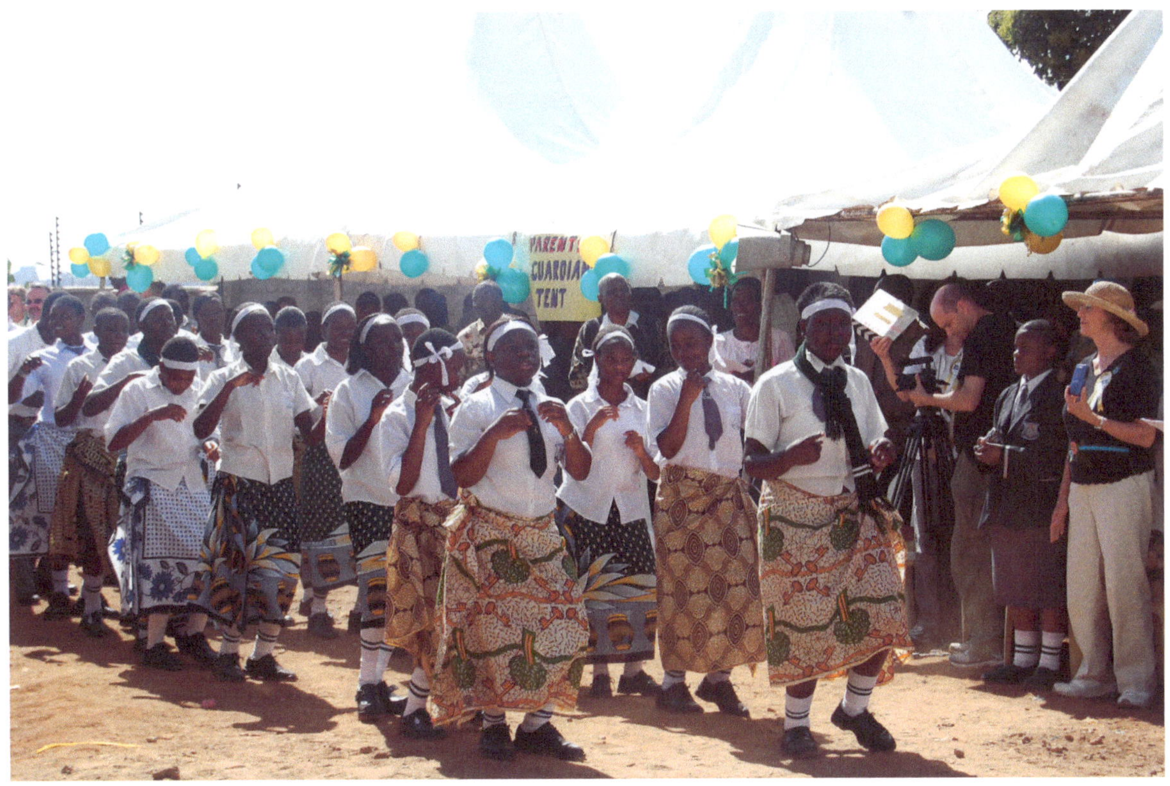

Students participate in the celebratory mass marking the opening of the new school.

St. Aloysius Gonzaga
Sec. School
GRAND OPENING OF ST. ALOYSIUS
GONZAGA SECONDARY SCHOOL
ON 20TH JUNE 2010

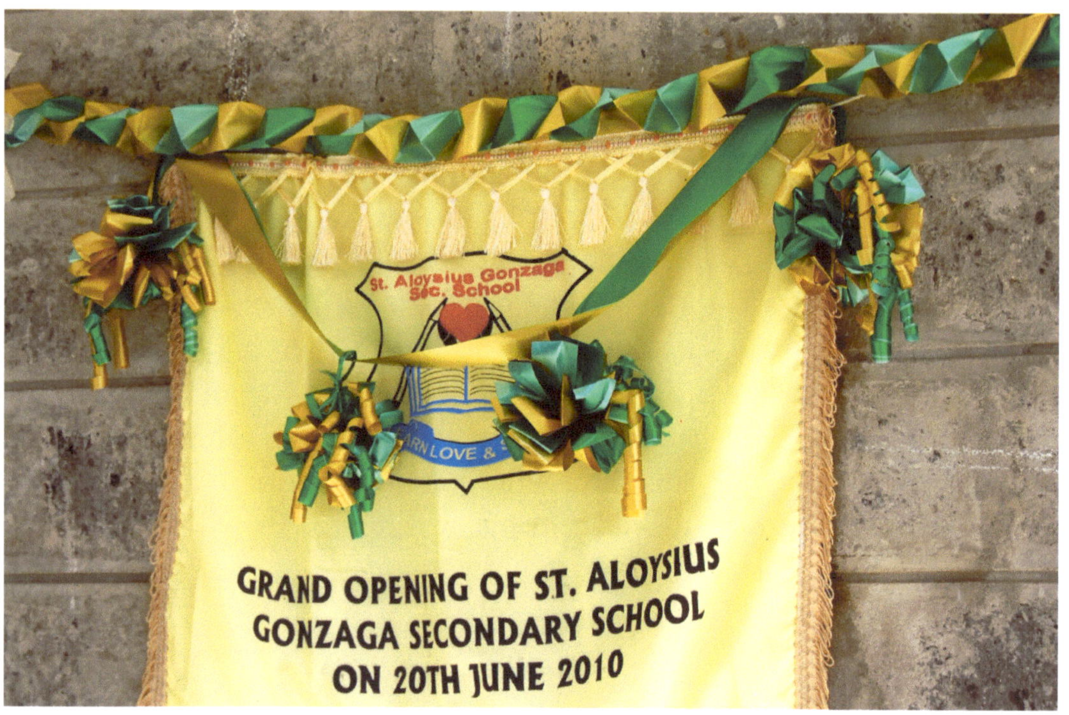

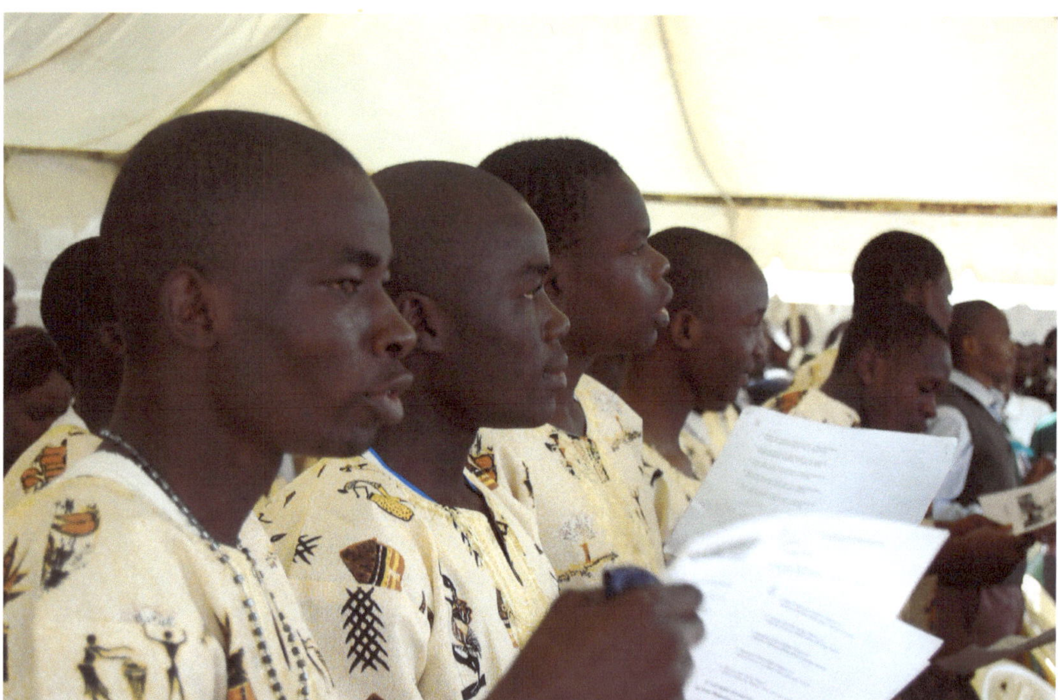

Singing during the celebratory mass.

The celebration mass of St. Aloysius Gonzaga was beautiful and, in true Kenyan fashion, long. Many speeches, I think eleven baptisms and many recognitions. Georgetown University was recognized for its contributions to the school with special mention of Phil Boroughs, Martha and Dave Swanson. Margaret and I were humbled to also receive thanks and recognition and were asked, along with all the Georgetown visitors, to come up in front of the nearly 700 people who were there to be recognized. I think Margaret and I learn as much, if not more, from delivering the Art in Kibera program than the students do. The reciprocity alone is overwhelming, then to have the founder of the school recognize us and have an art room?! It is simply overwhelming.

The irony is that, in my opinion, today was really about Phil and he was unable to attend the celebration because he was feeling ill. He is, however, on the mend and was able to go to the dinner. It was Phil that first introduced the school to all of us and, even though our 2007 Kenyan Immersion was not specifically about St. Al's for Margaret or me, it became the place we wanted to impact. It was really

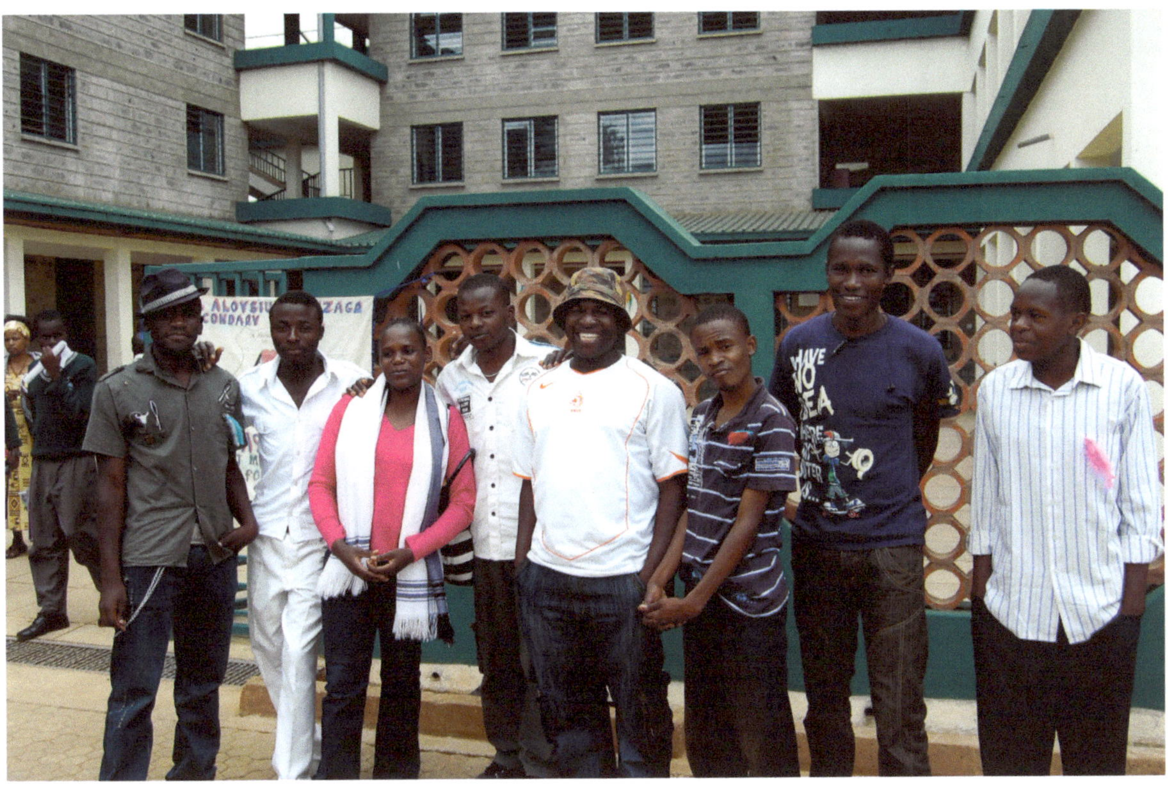

David Dinda and friends gather in front of St. Al's.

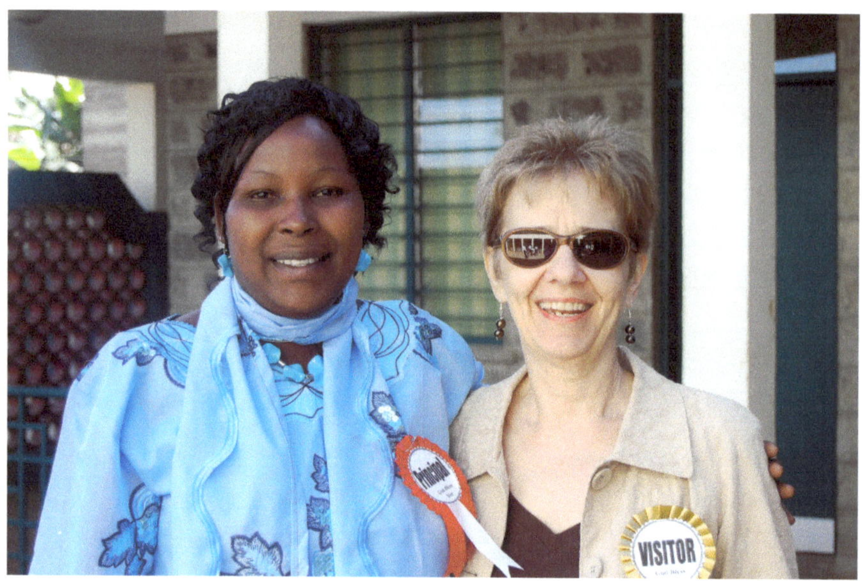

St. Al's Principal Beatrice and Margaret Halpin.

unfortunate that he couldn't be at today's mass, given all his efforts to make this dream a reality; however, he was recognized and thanked at every opportunity.

My Kenyan son, David Dinda, was there today and I was so excited to see him. We'll be spending a fair amount of time with him during the coming weeks. I am so proud of him; he has created the Foundation of Hope and they are doing great things in the Kibera slum to help others (more to come in this in a future blog). His foundation has taken over the space occupied by the old school so that space will not be gone to us, just repurposed with a new soul.

We spent the afternoon lunching with the 2010 Kenyan Immersion Group and then headed to dinner at Osteria to celebrate with what seemed like 100+ people. It was also great to see Dave and Martha Swanson again and realize that our worlds expand way past the Georgetown community and the gates of the University.

Tomorrow is our first day of classes and Margaret and I have never been more inspired. It is so amazing to see how our students are prospering. They were selling their art today and were beyond excited about what they are going to do in Art Club. To be a part of this institution and legacy? We are honored.

Much Love and be well,

Charles and Margaret

MONDAY, JUNE 21, 2010

The first day of year three. We are off and running.

We started our day at the Kuona Trust Art Centre which houses artists in residence, programs for artist development and a wonderful gallery that was used by the journalism club last year to display their photo journalism exhibit. If all goes as planned, we'll be having an art exhibit here this Friday. It is exciting to think that these artists will be displaying their art for public view for the first time in their lives. What an opportunity for these smart, beautiful and important students. They make our hearts full.

We arrived early at the school, and it was a good thing that we did as they had not alerted the students as to when or how we'll be starting this year; so there was

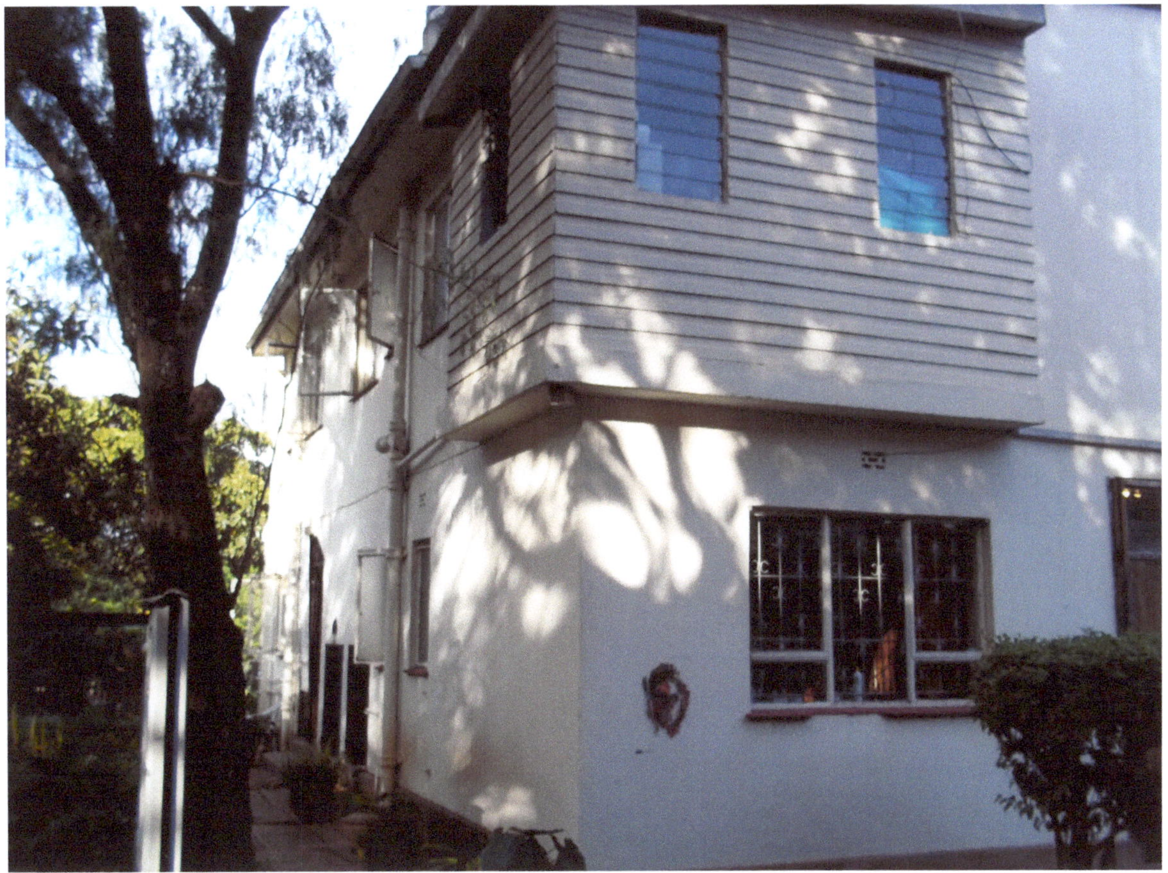

Kuona Trust Centre for Visual Arts.

a lot of running around. New school or not, the wise words of Phil Boroughs remain true: "It will never go as planned." Because of the shuffle and getting the students prepared to meet with us, Margaret and I met jointly with the students from Forms 1 through 4 to explain what we will be doing. We went over the new curriculum, talked about our expectations, talked about the exhibit and also got them prepared for lots of work. We asked if there were questions and one student asked about the photos they took three years ago and about different elements we had taught in previous sessions. It is amazing that it has all stuck with them. We have also learned that some of our students have gone off to the Buruburu Institute of Fine Arts in Kenya and one is a working artist. Who knew?

We came back to Pedro Arrupe for some light exercise and a pleasant dinner with a bunch of Jesuits and a nun. As always, it was great.

Tomorrow will truly be a day of art practice and working with the students.

Be well and thanks for following us,

Charles and Margaret

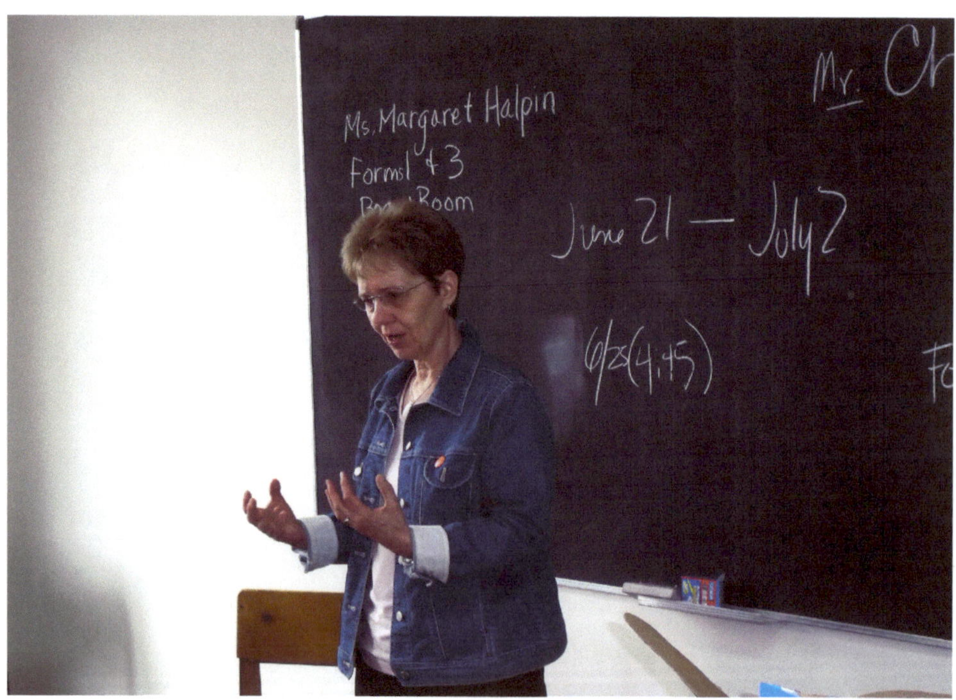

Margaret passionately delivers the art curriculum.

TUESDAY, JUNE 22, 2010

A day of contrasts and rewards.

I write this in a state of exhaustion. Today was a long one and it's only 8:30 pm. We started at David Dinda's Foundation of Hope in St. Al's old Kibera location. I know I said that we would miss the place and the familiar walk to the school. I was reminded today that it's really all about the students and now that the students have moved, the walk down to the old school from the street is harsh, a grim reminder of the squalor and everyday realities that are part and parcel of Kibera. After the visit, Margaret and I agreed that we don't miss that location at all. The source of our joy and passion is the students and now that they are housed in a

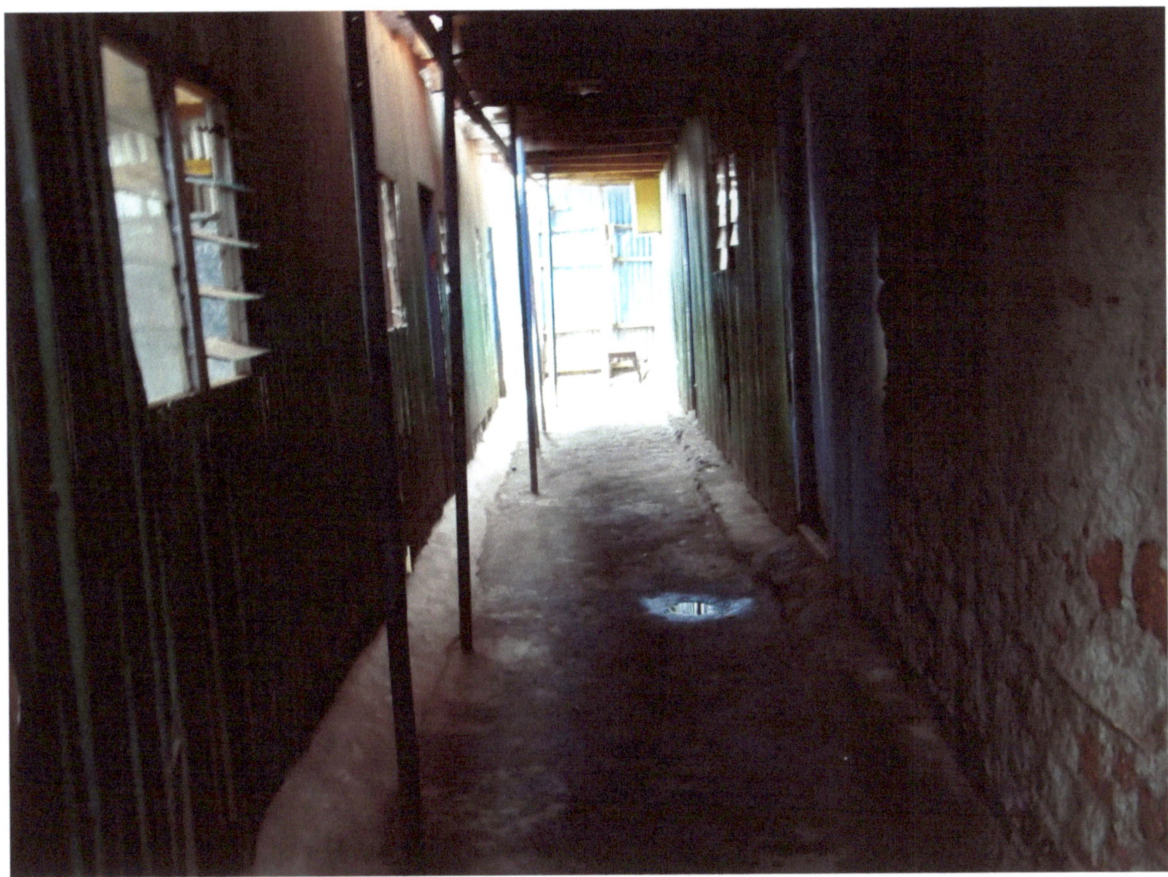

The empty halls of the old St. Al's school.

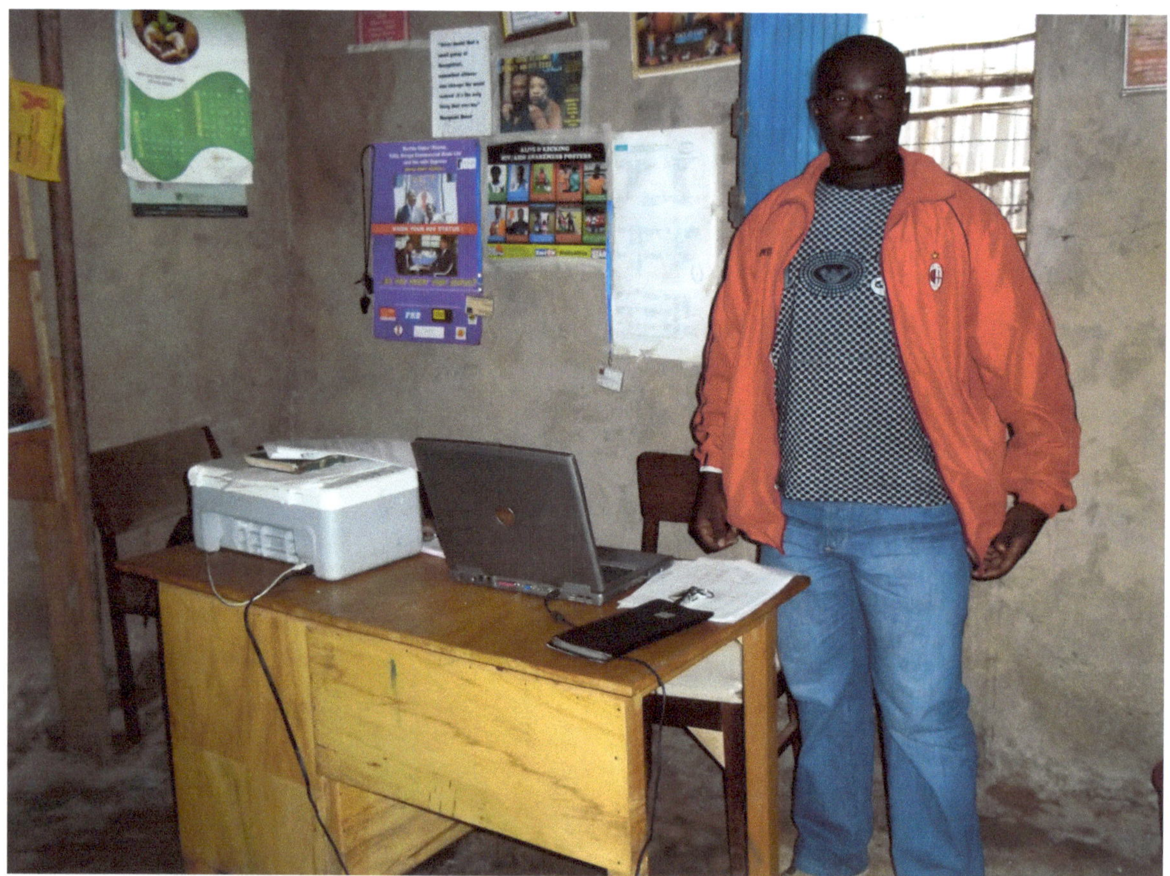

David Dinda's office at the new Foundation of Hope location.

new location, so is our excitement. In no way does this mean the re-purposing of the location for the Foundation of Hope isn't great; it really does fill an important need in the midst of the community it serves. However, as prior occupants, it almost makes it impossible to look back at the old school as an option once you have been in the new school.

We visited David's sister, Caroline, who has a strong connection to Margaret. A few years ago, Margaret purchased her a sewing machine to support her education as a seamstress; today, when we went to visit her at the shop/school where she learns/works, Margaret was presented with the gift of a beautiful dress that Caroline had made. It was just amazing and Margaret was so touched.

After lunch we were off and running at the new school. We now have two great rooms in which to teach. These children are even more attentive and engrossed now that we are in a classroom that is appropriately sized where we can actually

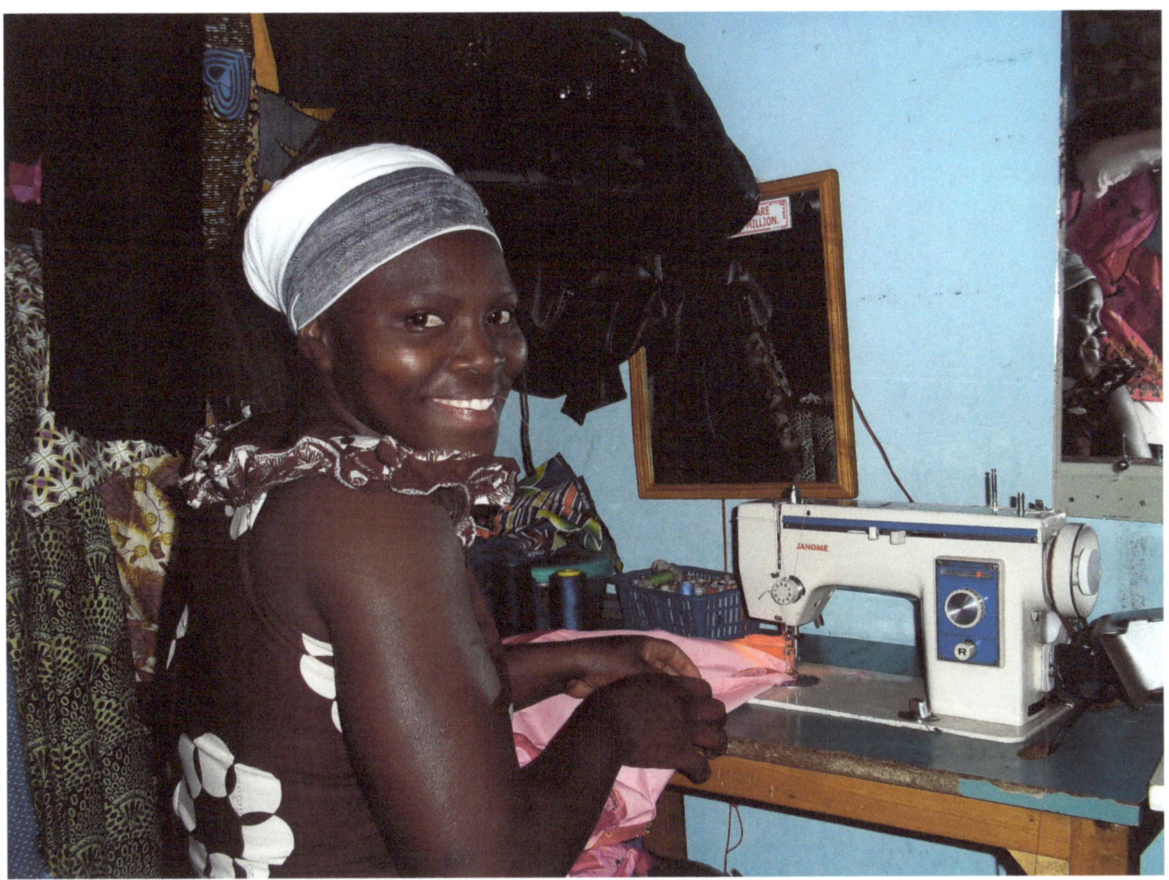

Caroline Dinda at her sewing machine.

be close to them. Before, due to the compactness of the rooms, we didn't have the ability to be right next to them or to gather everyone together for discussions.

Today our first classes were with Forms 3 and 4. Since they started the same year, they have the same curriculum and we wanted to talk to all of them about the upcoming exhibition, the new mediums we'll be using and the peace theme for this year's projects. We talked about what peace means, read quotes and engaged them in a conversation. You can see the wheels turning and the questions they asked were remarkable. For example, Collins asked if art depicting war could be representative of how one sometimes fights to gain, or maintain, peace. Wow. We also talked about peace between humans and governments. They went away with a lot to think about before they start creating art around the theme of peace. Our next classes were taught separately; I had Form 2 and Margaret had a new set of Form 1 students. Some of the kids already had some familiarity of the western

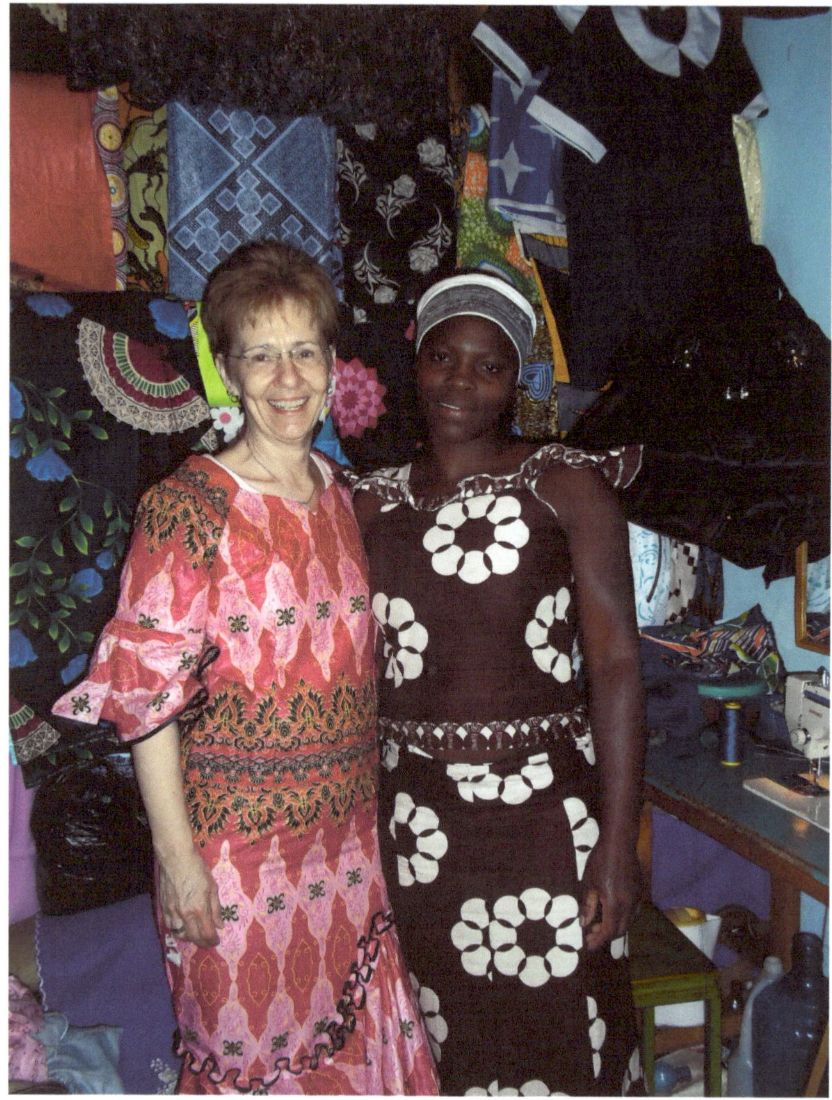

Margaret models her new dress.

artists and were able to talk about them based on the materials that had been left at the school or what they had heard from older students. Very encouraging!

We are off to go work on the gallery show, lesson plans and all the other things we need to do before we teach tomorrow afternoon.

Be well and thanks for following us on this journey.

Charles and Margaret

WEDNESDAY, JUNE 23, 2010

Day Three.

Everything is running smoothly and the art program will be having its first Gallery Exhibition at the Kuona Trust Art Centre this Friday. All the preparations have been made for this group's first ever, honest-to-goodness art exhibition. It's the real deal. As you can imagine, we're very excited. Today was filled with intense work as we discovered there is no stock of art for the show!!!! At the event last week, the art club sold ALL of their art. I guess that is both the good news and the bad news; now they have to make enough art in the next few days to be able to show on Friday. The Nation, the Standard and Reuters were all invited, so these kids might get some press.

The students were quiet today as they focused on their work. I played classical music as they painted. Margaret's classes were quiet as well and, although they did

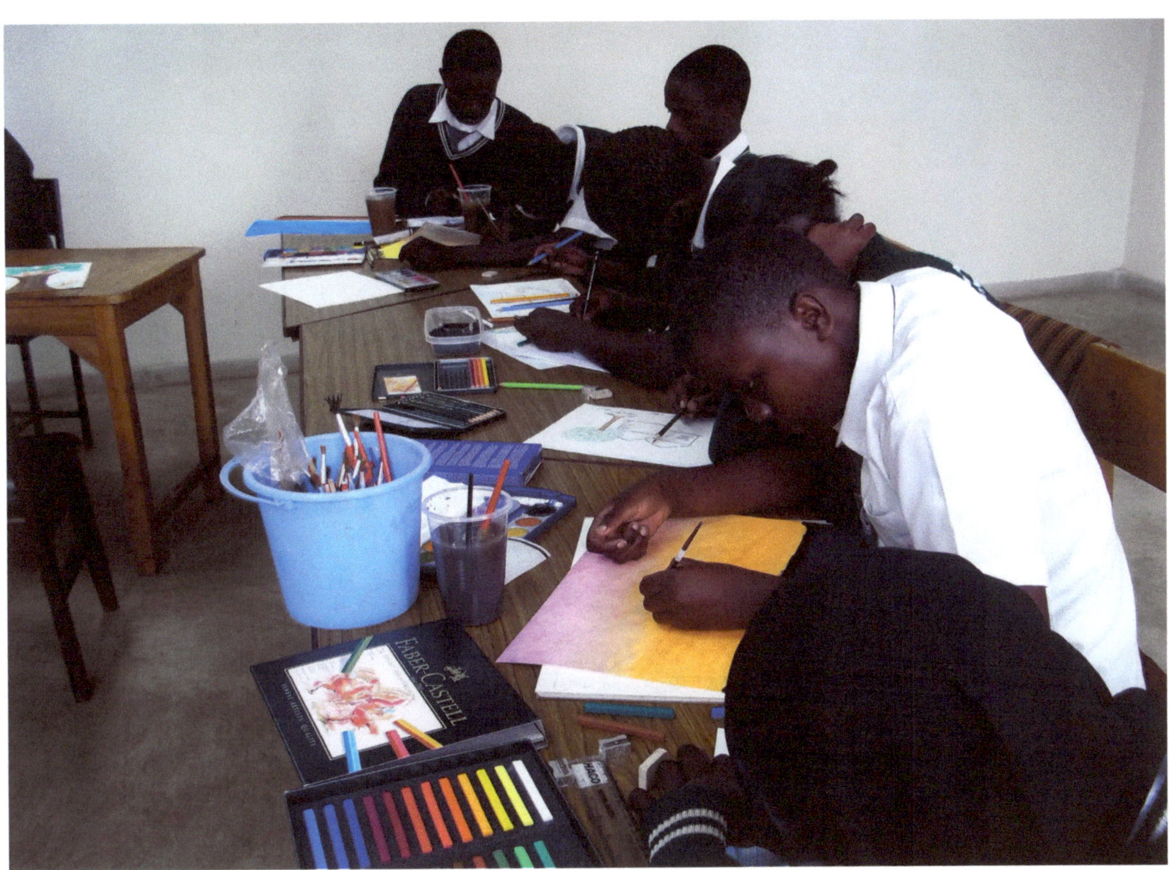

not listen to classical tunes, they were listening to a performance in the assembly room that was echoing down the hall. Once this art program really starts moving each year, it seems to have a life of its own.

We had dinner back at the community with the Jesuits and Sr. Mary Owens, head of Nyumbani. We then spent time with the Georgetown 2010 group on their last evening in Kenya. It is very nice having them all here and we hope to have a meal with them tomorrow before they depart.

Not much more to add other than to say that it's exciting to do this work and we're happy that you are on this journey with us.

Be well,

Charles and Margaret

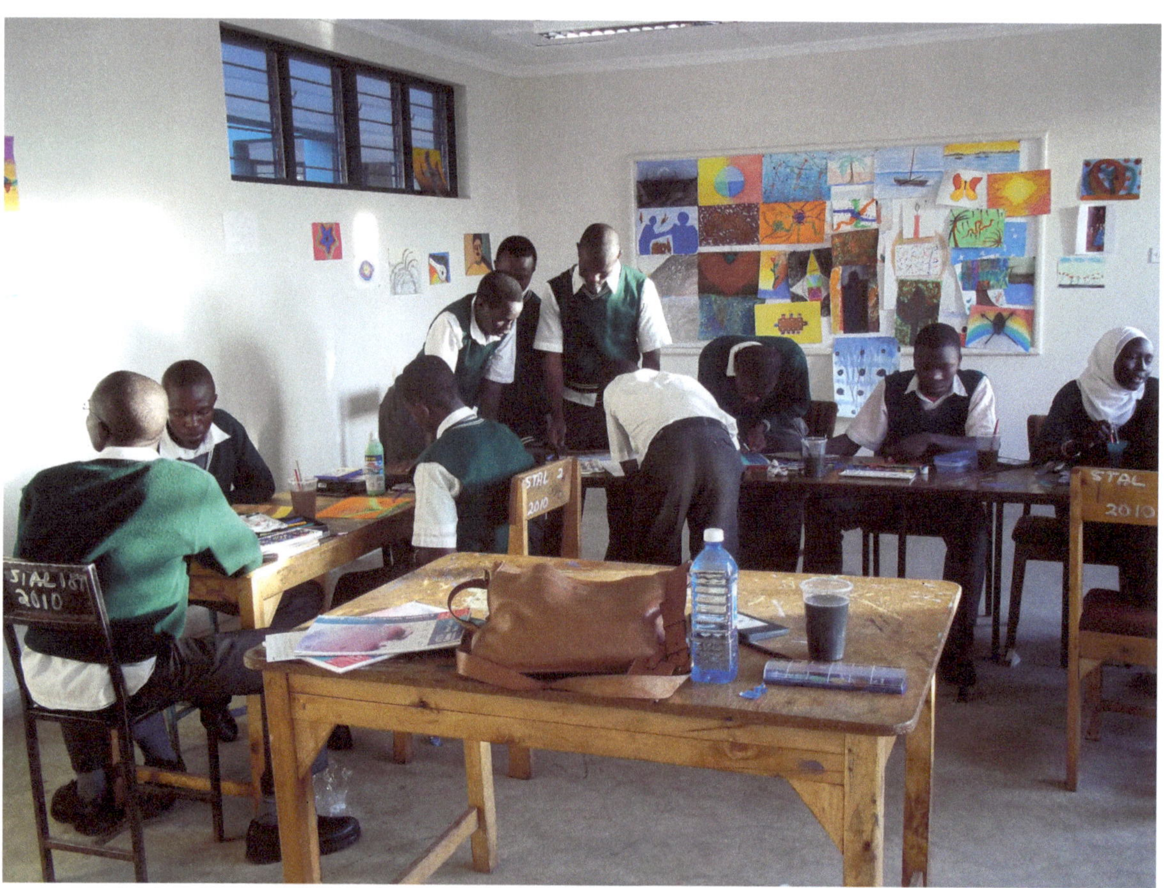

Students prepare for the upcoming art exhibit.

Below is the announcement for the art exhibition:

kuona trust
centre for visual arts

Likoni Close, Likoni Lane, off Dennis Pritt Road, Hurlingham

PO Box 4802, Nyayo Stadium 00506

Tel: (254) 0202405960 Mobile: 0721 262326, 0733 742752

Artists of St. Aloysius Gonzaga Secondary School Exhibition

Opening 25th June 2010 at 6.30 pm

St. Aloysius Gonzaga, is a Catholic secondary school that serves HIV/AIDS affected young people from the Kibera slums in Nairobi, Kenya.

On an initial visit, Georgetown University administrators realizing the absence of a visual art education, created an art immersion program. These artists receive art instruction annually from these administrators who first visited Kibera in 2007. After the first year of this art immersion program the artists/students formed the art club which functions all year around with the intensive art instruction delivered in a two-week annual art immersion program for those students interested in art.

In its 3rd year, the art immersion program has yielded some amazing artists that know how to convey their talent as well as their story about the place they live, the Kibera slum here in Nairobi, Kenya.

This has resulted in a successful body of work that really represents the fantastic art ability of the smart, beautiful and important students of St. Aloysius which has recently opened its new site in Lang'ata.

Please join us for this exhibition at the Kuona Trust, Centre for Visual Arts, Likoni Close, Likoni Lane off Dennis Pritt Rd, Hurlingham on Friday**, June 25th, 2010 at 6:30 pm** for the opening of the "Artists of St. Aloysius Gonzaga Secondary School". The show will be open through **27th June 2010**.

RSVP: Kuona Trust or Charles DeSantis, Georgetown University
Tel. 0718767077

THURSDAY, JUNE 24, 2010

It just keeps getting better and better.

Today began with the wonderful sound of Deborah Moijoi knocking on my guest house door. It feels like home here. Deborah is an important piece of coming home to Pedro Arrupe and Nairobi; and now part of coming home will include Joseph, her beautiful 7 month-old. He has captured my heart. Wow, and if he doesn't look like a Moijoi, I don't know who does.

Today Margaret and I had lunch with the Kenya Immersion group at the Vernadah and dinner with them at Talisman. It was such a wonderful experience for Margaret and I to have Georgetown friends here in our special place. I really want to thank Phil for always being so inclusive and creating that feeling of community

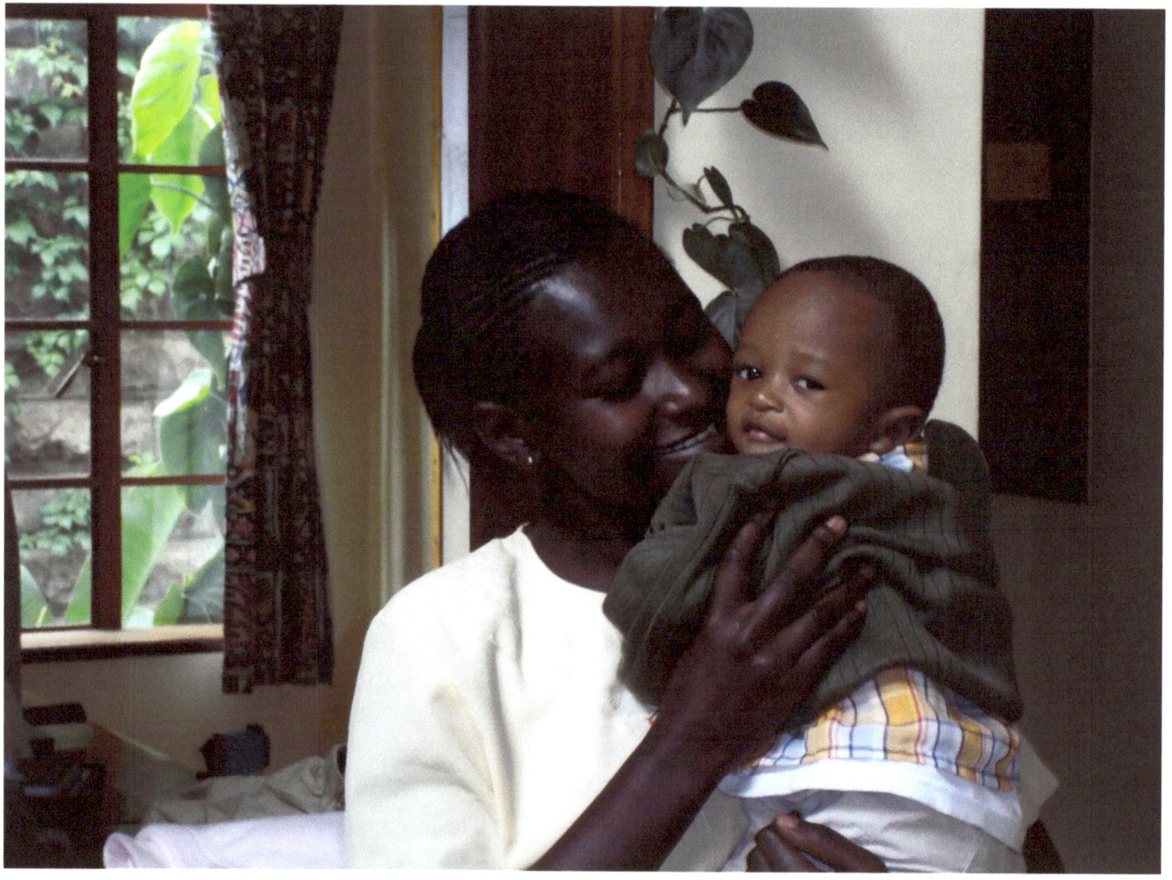

Deborah and Joseph Moijoi.

that is so distinctly Georgetown regardless of whether you are in Washington, Qatar, or in this case, Nairobi.

I am pleased to say that we have the art we need for the exhibition. It is a good thing too, because tomorrow the press, 54 students and 4 administrators from St. Al's will be attending an Art Exhibit complete with reception and an introduction of our smart, beautiful and important artists. Can you believe it? I can't.

Today the students showed up 1/2 hour early for class. I didn't question why they were so early (and not in another class); I was just glad they were there and ready. My Form 4 class was spectacular. We were listening to classical again and Castro, one of the artists, said to me "It's beautiful but not very interesting." I said that I was more interested in him connecting to and creating his art and not being distracted by the music. His response, after a very brief moment of contemplation, was "Good point." We walked away with a bunch of art and a lot to do tomorrow to

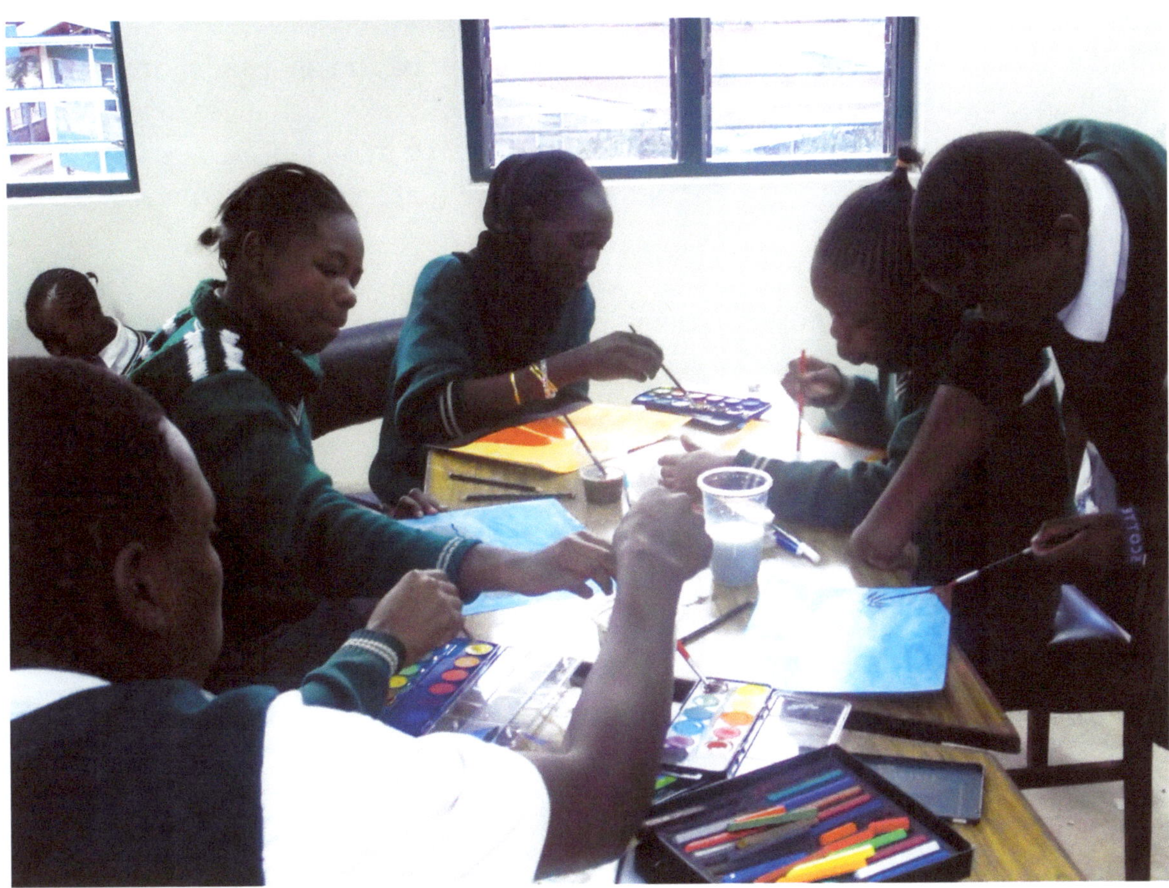

—as they say in the industry— "hang" this show. Thank God that during Margaret's twelve years of teaching art she put together as many student shows. Margaret's class has created some really different and wonderful pieces. They are talented. Her Form 1 class hangs on to her every word; it's great to see how attentive they are. We still can't believe how these kids soak up their art education. They get it, they get it, they get it.... Wow, I wish we had more to give.

Tonight's dinner with the Georgetown group was fun although they were in a bit of frenzy to make it to the airport on time. Traveling in large groups has its complexities. Margaret and I came a little late, the group left, then we finished our dinner and split a desert while talking about how rewarding and yet familiar it feels to be teaching in Kenya; particularly how nice it is to be teaching students who want to be taught. The work is hard, rewarding, restorative, refreshing, reflective and motivating for us. I can't believe that as hard as it feels to tear ourselves away from our normal lives, we get to be here doing something that gives so much to both our student artists and to us.

It is all about reciprocity. It is all about relationships and sharing your passions; it's all about going outside of your comfort zone and taking chances; it's all about believing in yourself and knowing that others believe in us too.

The next blog entry will be about the Art Exhibit at the Kuona Trust Center for Visual Arts.....

Thank you for your support and being on this journey with us.

Charles and Margaret

FRIDAY, JUNE 25, 2010

Art Exhibit at the Kuona Trust Centre for Visual Arts.

Although we're exhausted, we cannot sleep until we share our incredible experience with you. This morning I stopped by the office of St. Al's Principal, Beatrice, to pick up a few last pieces of art for the show. She and another faculty member commented that now that they have continued to see this impressive display of talent, they're wondering if they should appeal to the Ministry of Education to have Art included in the core curriculum at the school. I was speechless, but also in a hurry because Margaret and I needed to "hang the show" at Kuona Trust. Wow, to think that our art program may change the format of the curriculum for St. Al's. I can't believe it.

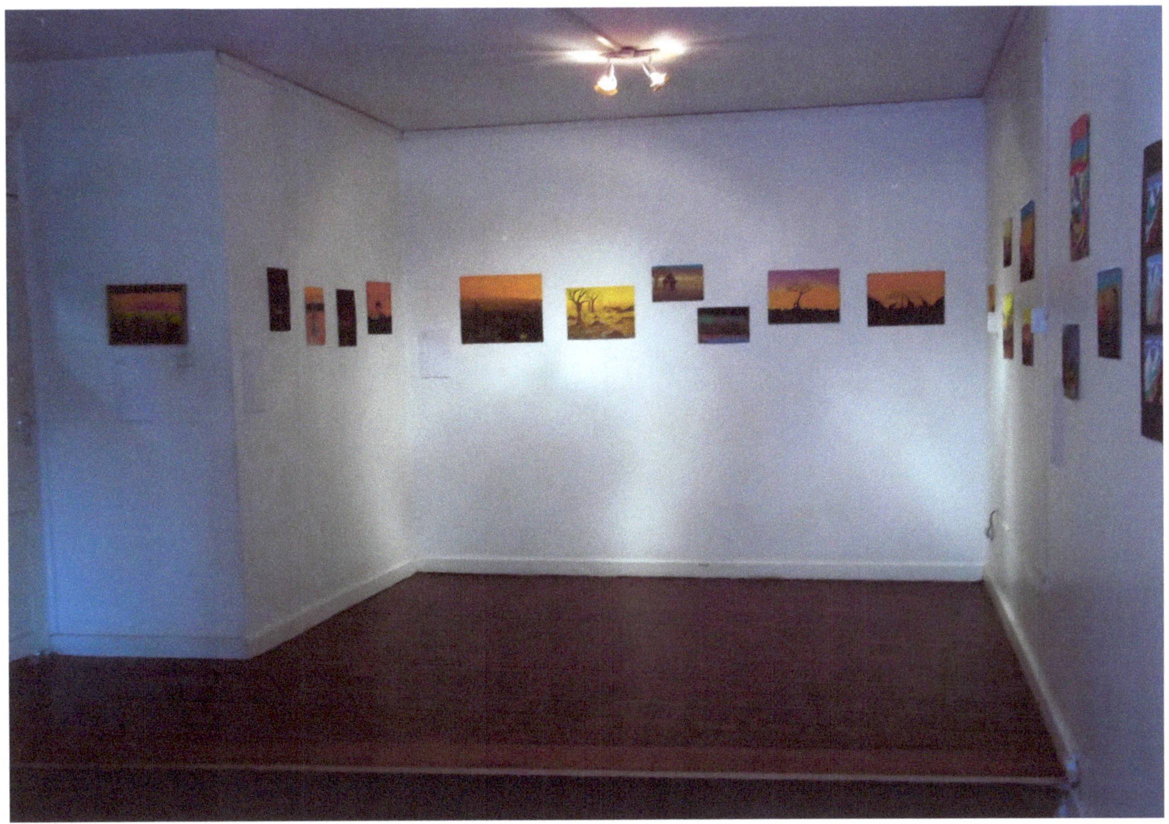

The art has been hung for the student art exhibition.

After grabbing a quick lunch, Margaret and I had our work cut out for us. Based on Margaret's experience, hanging the show was going to be her gig. She basically laid out all the art in the gallery and grouped it together; while she was doing this, I was creating and working with Kuona Trust's Head of School Programs to create the program that would be distributed. This meant getting the names of the artists matched with their work so that everyone gets the recognition they so deeply deserve.

We were done with only two hours to spare. Then they closed the gallery to clean it before the show. This was the real deal and it was great to see not only how important this is to our students and those of us affiliated with St. Al's, but how important it is to Thom at Kuona Trust. So, as the magic hour approached, Margaret changed into a delightful outfit, I put on a bowtie and sports coat and we were set.

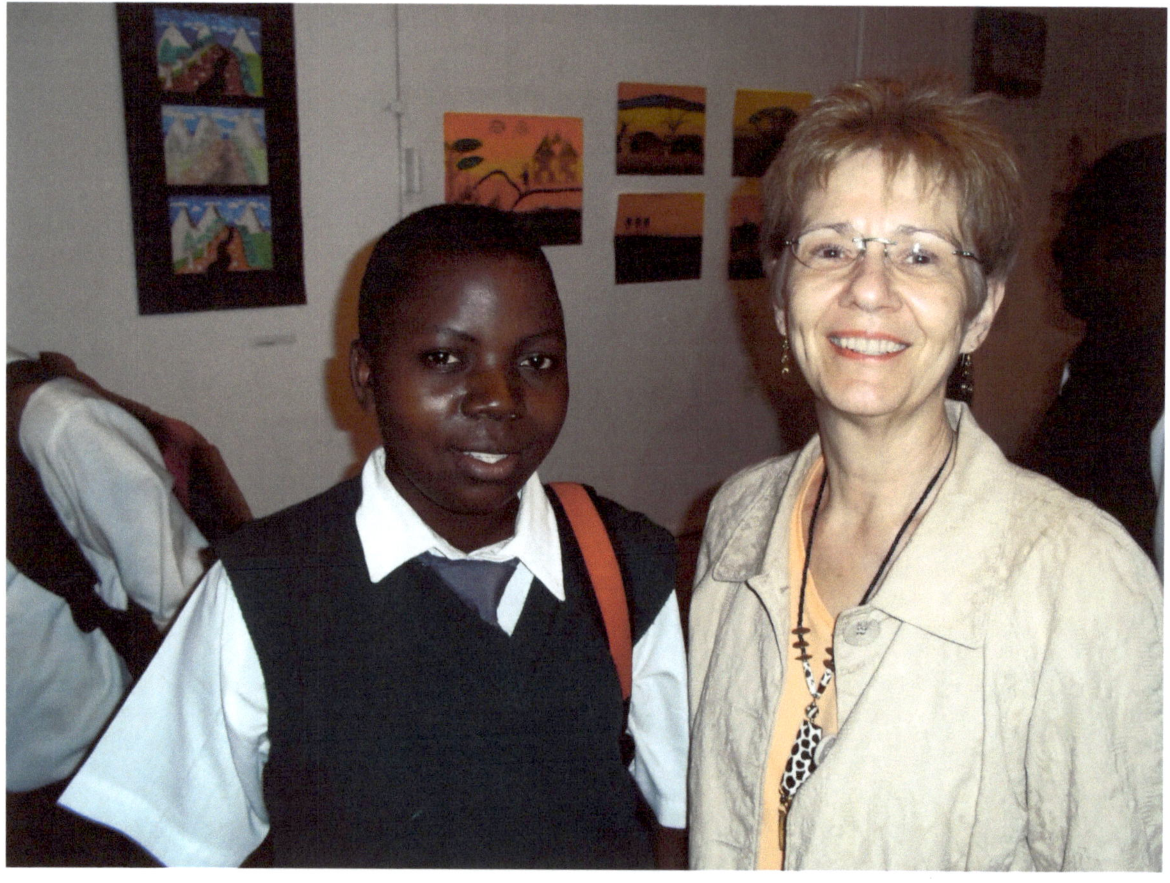

Margaret and student enjoy the show.

Okay, so as you may recall from last year's blog, there is Kenyan Time and then there's traffic. The bus left the school at 5 pm and didn't arrive across town until 7:05 pm. The traffic during peak commute time is horrible, add Friday to the mix and it is really bad. While we waited, one of our guests, Sr. Mary Owens, executive director of Nyumbani Home for AIDS orphans in Kenya, arrived. I am on the Board of Directors of this organization and was so happy that Mary came to support us.

We shook hands with each of the students, faculty and staff as they entered the grounds; Margaret and I started this tradition during our first year of teaching when we would stand outside our classroom and greet each student by shaking their hand. As they filled the gallery there was noise and excitement and picture taking with a lot of ooohs and ahhhhs and asking the principal to come look at this or to have a picture taken with their work. It was a level of excitement I hadn't seen

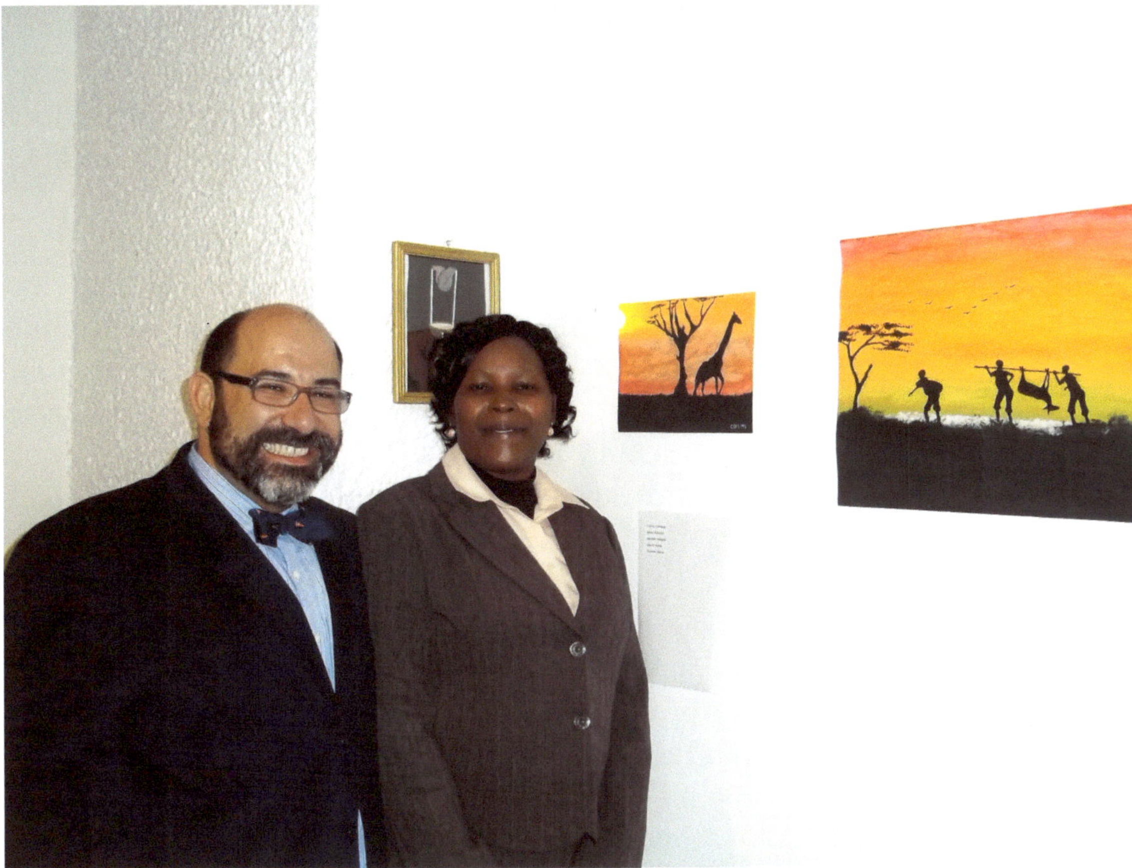

Charles with St. Al's Principal, Beatrice.

before. It was such a powerful and emotional moment; I looked over at Margaret, and in just a quick glance I could tell she was experiencing the exact same thing. We felt like the work that we came to do with this program had been realized. I was, and am still, in shock. Impressed and proud does not truly capture the feelings that Margaret and I were experiencing but it's all I can come up with.

Margaret asked me to represent us in a speech to the group. I enjoyed being able to thank everyone for all that they do to realize such great art and to remind them that our whole reason for coming each year is to be with these smart, beautiful and important people that we love and admire. In true Kenyan fashion, immediately following my speech, the power went out.

Power or no power, we carried on. People were taking pictures in the dark, eating food outside and walking around enjoying themselves; they didn't care a bit that the power was out. As we were all gathered eating food, drinking soda (wine for the adults) and taking in the event, Sarah, Jamie and Consuelo from Georgetown's Masters in Conflict Resolution program showed up. After explaining that the power was out, we grabbed a candle and toured them through the show. They loved it and all the students loved them. They grabbed a glass of wine, took it all in and hung out with the students. It was just great. It has been nice to share this with so many people that we are connected with in DC.

As we loaded everyone back onto the bus to return the student artists to their homes, the lights came back on. As always, nothing goes as you expect it to in Kenya. We all laughed. Two very important developments came out of this evening's event: 1) Thom and Patrick of Kuona Trust are committed to partnering with us on this show annually and 2) I believe in the coming years, art will be included as part of the official curriculum at St. Al's.

St. Al's Principal, Beatrice, and two of its faculty members, Bernard and John, joined us on the ride home because they do not live in Kibera which is where the bus was returning the students. I thanked them for coming and allowing us to deliver this program. Beatrice looked at me and said, "We should be thanking you. The sacrifice you and Margaret make is what makes this a success." Not once in the three years of delivering this program would I have characterized any element of this as a sacrifice. None of it. I asked Margaret and she said not at all. Maybe we have to work here with the program and still tend to our responsibilities at Georgetown or have difficulty scheduling to get away, but sacrifice? Not at all. It is a gift. We get as much out of this as the students do, and on some days, more.

Charles and Margaret

MONDAY, JUNE 28, 2010

It is definitely a village.

The weekend was great. We held Saturday Studio at the school and had a good turn out for three hours of studio time. We returned to Pedro Arrupe for a little rest before Anne Wangari arrived from Dadaab to spend time with us. I went to mass at the Nyumbani Home with Sr. Mary and Anne while Margaret stayed home and had time to her self. I have to say, if every mass was like it is at Nyumbani, I think churches would be filled to the brim, with Catholics and non-Catholics alike. The kids make it special; they dance, they sing and it's all about them. It was nice to see all the kids as well as some old friends like Lloydie Zaiser who is from the DC area and hosts Kenyan Education Service Trips. After mass, we relaxed at Pedro Arrupe and then went to take down the art exhibit and then to dinner. It was a nice Sunday.

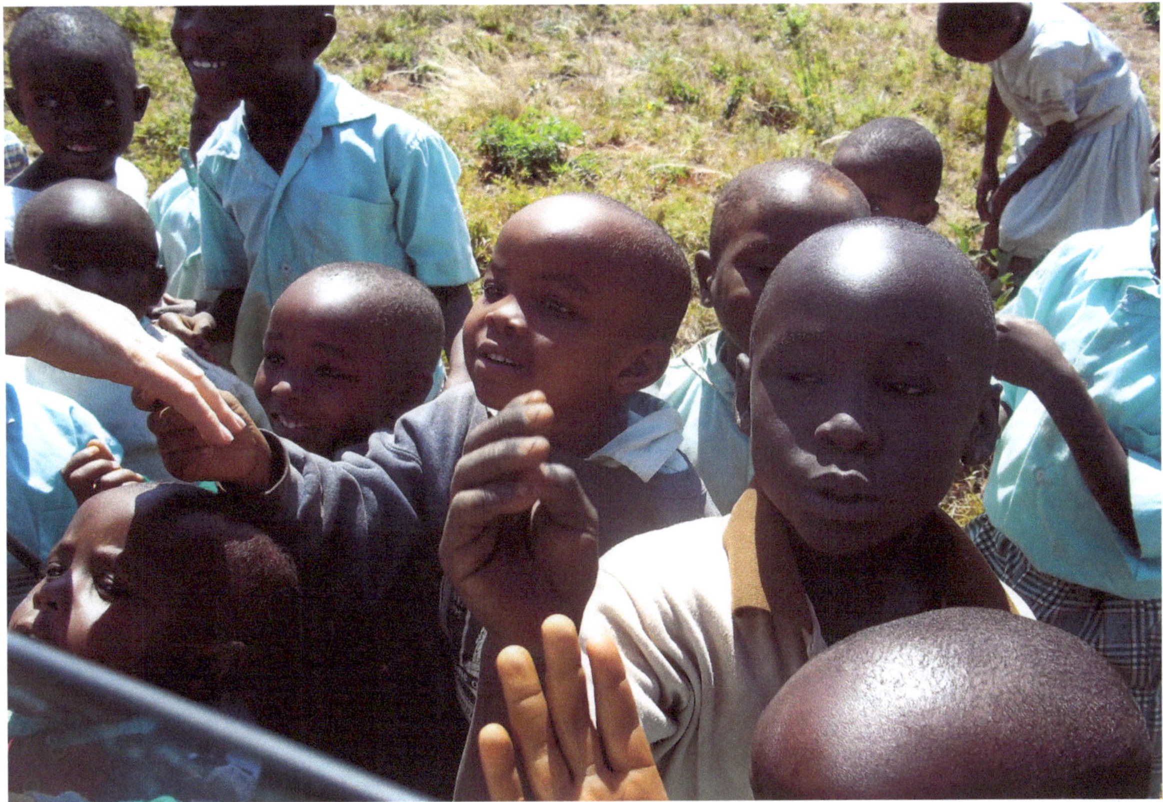

The children of Nyumbani Village.

Today, Monday, started at 6:15 am with a road trip to Kitui which is where the Nyumbani Village is located. The village is home to 663 AIDS orphan children and 64 grandparents that care for these kids. The village consists of homes made of interlocking brick, amazing schools, a clinic, a guest house, agriculture - you name it and it was there.

The model is grandparents and kids in a home with four homes on a block. I believe there are sixteen blocks in total. The melia trees are amazing and are what will, eventually, sustain the village. The melia is like a mahogany that can be harvested for hard wood furniture. There are 100 acres of it and it is growing well. The farms and the livestock were well cared for and the areas so clean; Nickolas, who has major oversight of the village, was great. The residents of the village speak little to no English but it all works out.

I was so impressed. As a Nyumbani Board Member, my feeling of pride for this organization just grew ten fold. Sr. Mary Owens is a rock star for leading this to the place it is today.

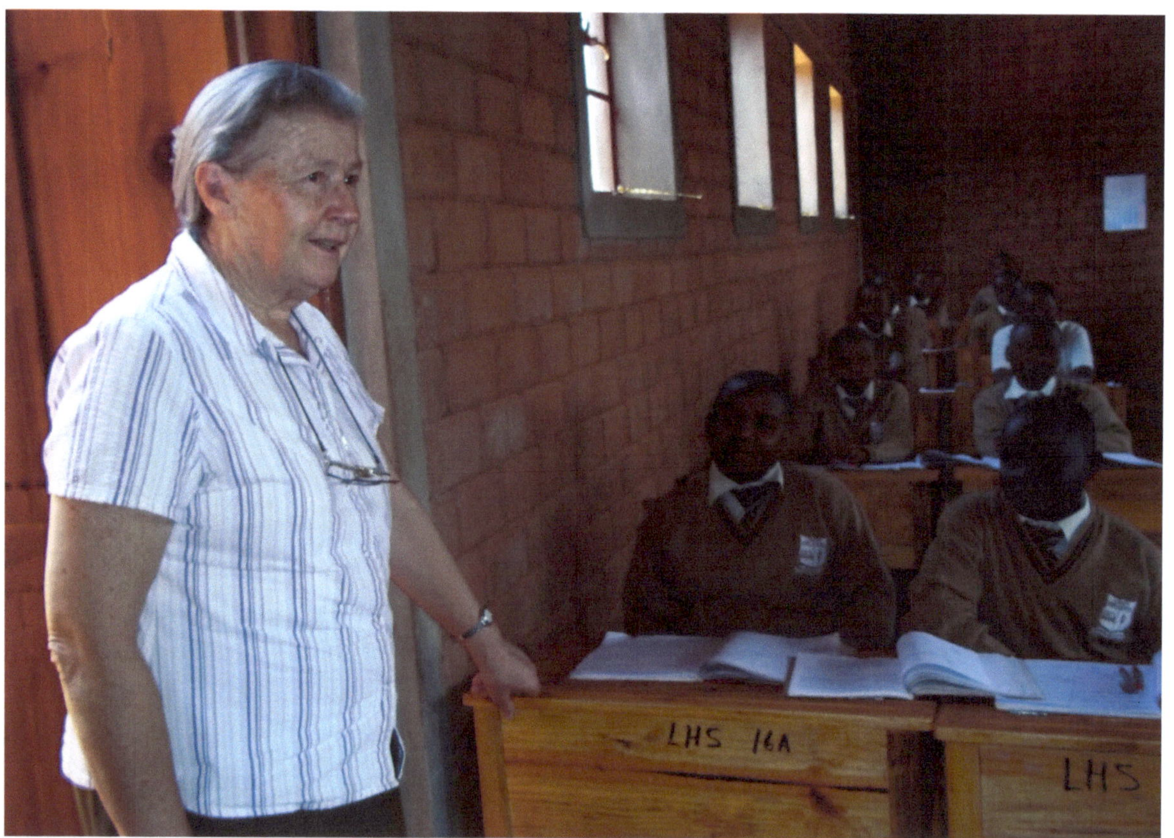

Sister Mary Owens, Executive Director of Nyumbani.

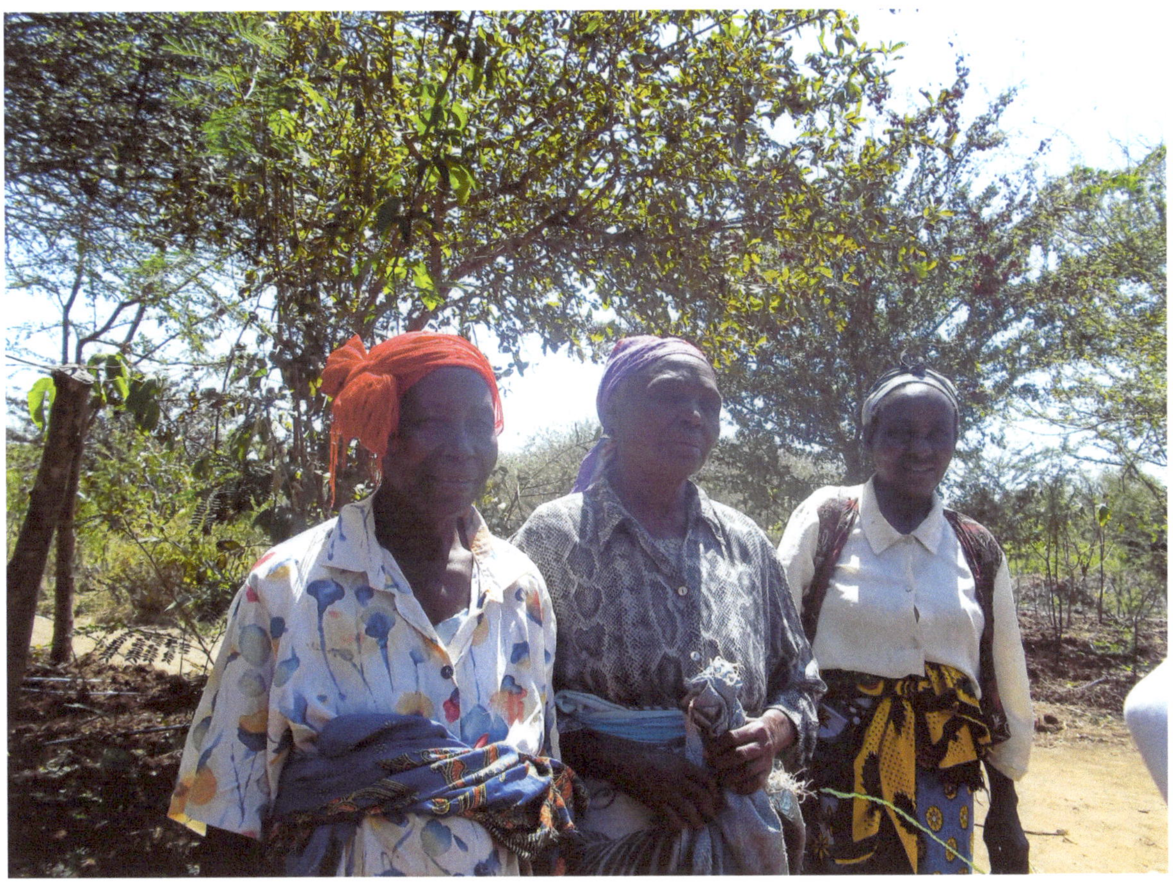

A trio of grandmothers from Nyumbani Village.

We left the village at 1pm to return to Nairobi in order to teach our 4:15 classes and we got back with time to spare. When you are on a schedule with Sr. Mary, you can be sure that it will be kept.

After a low key and rewarding class, we joined Anne for dinner where the three of us reflected on our day. I am exhausted and about to fall asleep but if I did not get this out, I might lose some of the details.

Be well and we appreciate you being on this journey with us.

Charles and Margaret

TUESDAY, JUNE 29, 2010

The school feels like it has a soul.

It's another beautiful day in Nairobi. I've noticed that every time I walk into St. Al's, it feels like more than just a building where students come to be educated, it feels like a place filled with soul. The movement of the students, the voices, the feelings, the impacts, the learning and the development. It definitely feels like it has a soul to me.

Today was supposed to be more of a lecture day with our primary topic being Frank Lloyd Wright. However, the projector for the laptop was not available so we moved onto painting instead. My first class is Form 4 and they are skillful

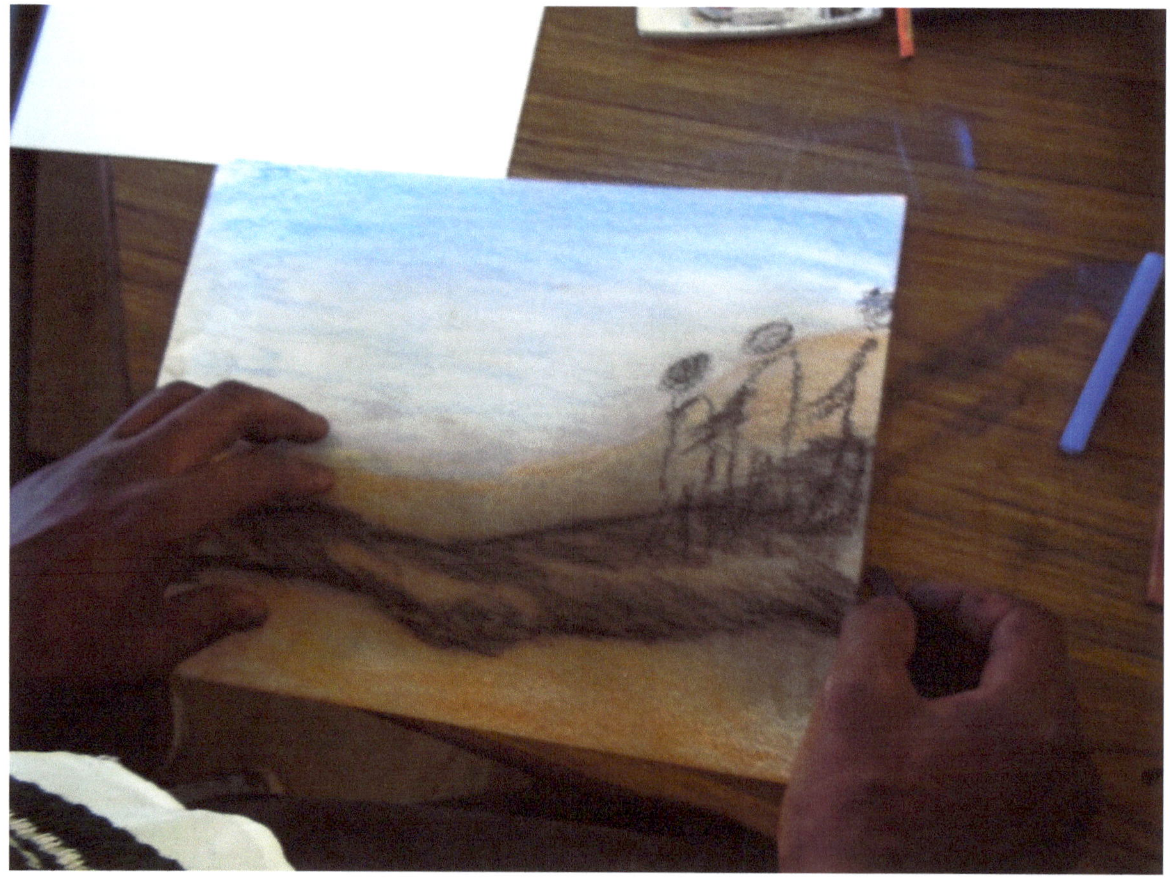

An artist in Form 4 steps out of their comfort zone.

painters who have really perfected the narrative of the Kibera slum and the Kenyan experience. Their skills continue to improve, but their subject matter hasn't shown much variation. After an hour, I spoke to them about how well they've done, how much they've learned and how similar everything they're producing looks. I urged them to consider breaking out of the box, allowing themselves to feel uneasy while they paint, and to try doing something that isn't representative of what they have perfected. I reminded them that they are smart, beautiful and important and with that comes a responsibility to keep reaching beyond what they've already achieved. There was not a bit of love for me after that speech. I could tell that they didn't want to hear that I wanted them to be different. I gave them some time to work and said, "Knock yourselves out. I'll see you in an hour."

I took my Form 2 class to one of the other available rooms for a history and drawing lesson. This group is always quiet, amenable and attentive. They are also very good at drawing. When I returned to Form 4, they had had a breakthrough. It was phenomenal. There were Rothkos and Pollacks and all these unique and unconstrained pieces of art. I asked them what the experience had felt like, and they all said it felt freeing. It nearly brought tears to my eyes. Art makes a difference in people's lives. The proof is in these students, in their attitudes and perspectives. Just then Margaret walked in, looked around the room and said to me, "They had a breakthrough." In moments like these I think of my dear friend, neighbor and colleague, Professor Tony Arend. He helps students have breakthroughs all the time. I can tell. I've experienced more than one breakthrough with him myself, during some of our intense conversations. Thank you for inspiring me, Tony.

Margaret's classes are doing well, working diligently and using color to wonderful effect, particularly one student, Saisi Wycliffe. And why shouldn't he be using great colors with a rock star artist name like Saisi Wycliffe? Who doesn't want a name like that? I do. Margaret's Form 1 class is really focused (unlike her first Form 1 group from 2008); and the Form 3 class is motivated and maturing. They really love Margaret's demeanor and look up to her. She is definitely a model teacher: focused, direct and open.

After class we met up with friends for a nice dinner at Talisman. The group included Anne Wangari and the students from the Masters in Conflict Resolution program. Connections were made as the Georgetown women may join Anne in Dadaab for a women's conference in July. It helps to be related to the Kenyan Anne Wangari. She is so wonderful and a world of help.

We have two more days of classes followed by our day of celebration then we leave Nairobi on Saturday. As always, I can't believe it has gone by so fast. It feels great to be here and I am inspired every day by the students and the amazing Kenyan people that we have connected with.

Assante Sana (thank you very much) for joining us on this Journey.

Charles and Margaret

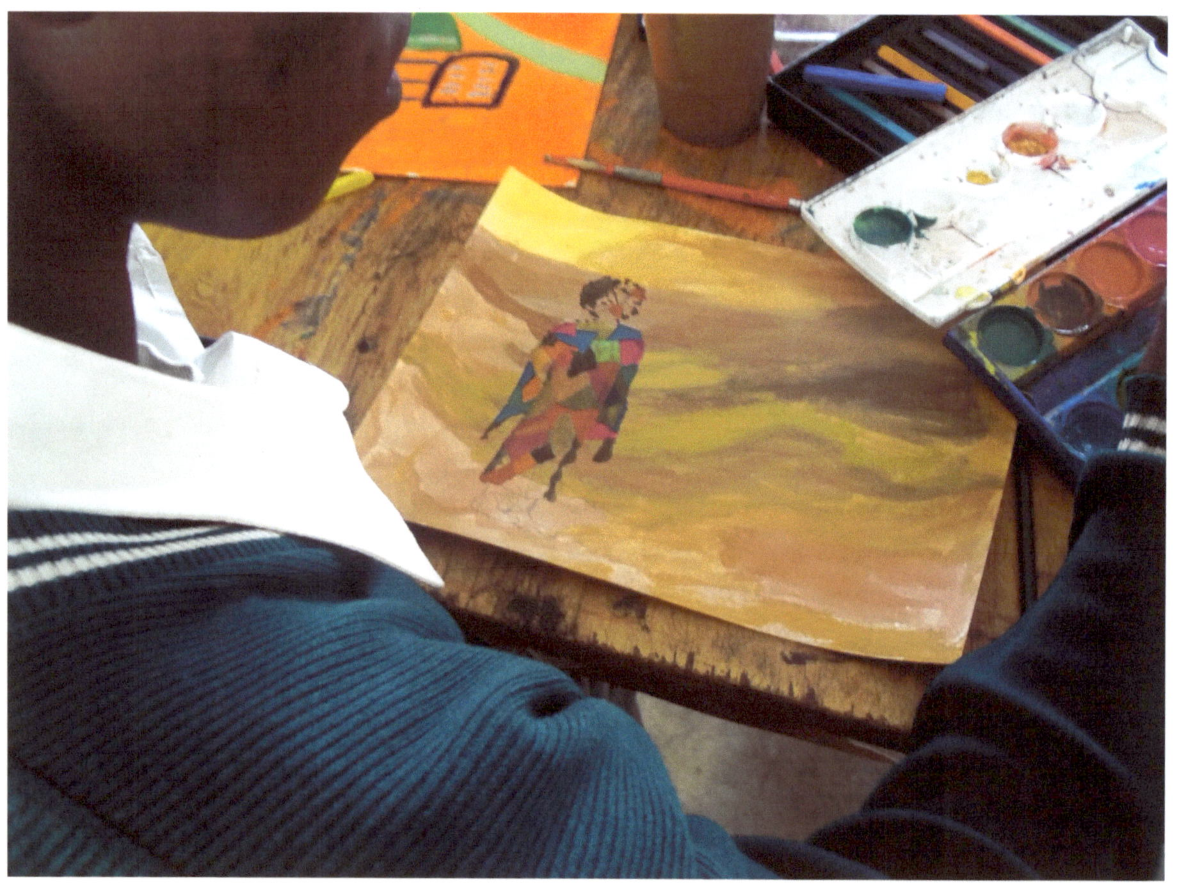

WEDNESDAY, JUNE 30, 2010

Art is in the air.

We went downtown to see our friends at the Text Book Centre to purchase more nice paper. Due to the timing of our classes, we've found ourselves dealing with commuter traffic, which is not fun at all. On several occasions we've been convinced that we'd be late for our classes but we always manage to pull it off. Today when I got to class, I continued to watch the Form 4 class blossom. I asked them why it took me telling them to go outside of their comfort zones for them to take some risks in their work. The answer was clear: the work that they've been exposed to through our classes has been largely literal. They also thought their work had to be

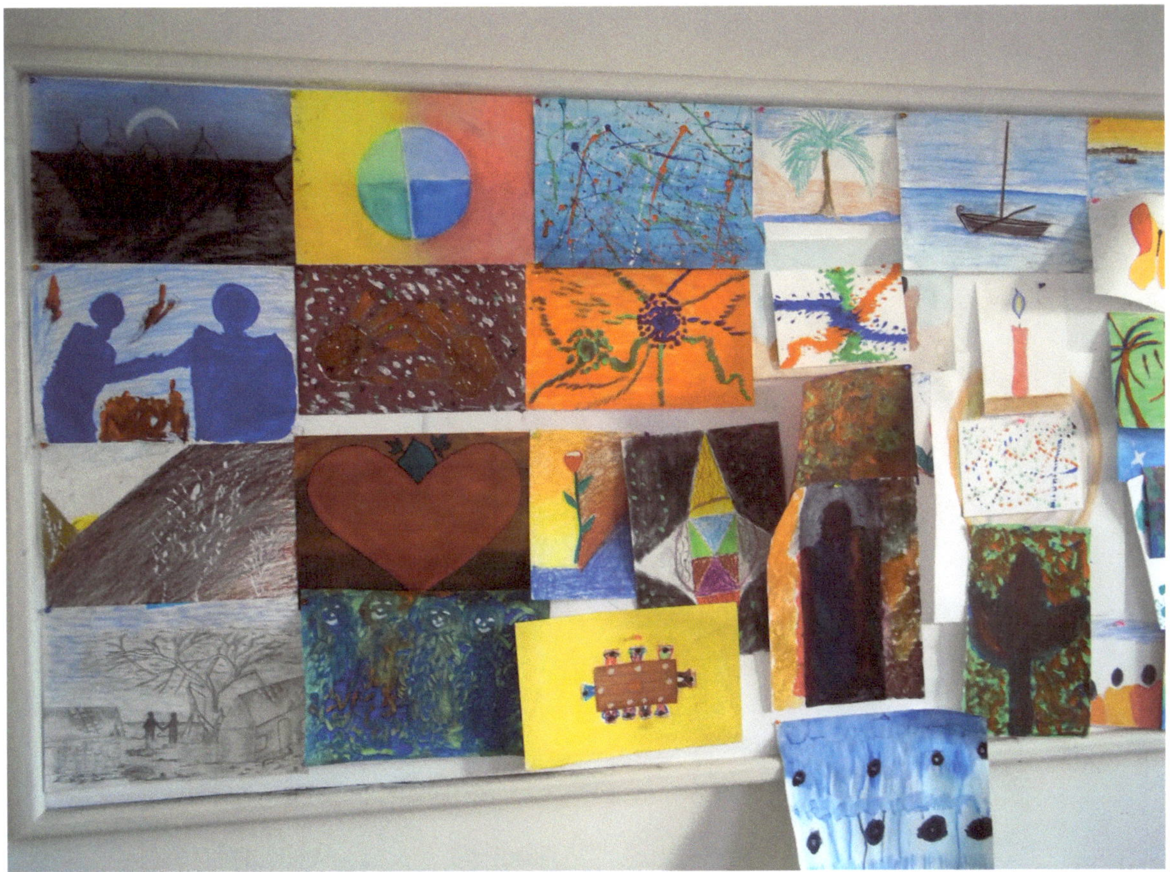

Breakthrough

recognizable by others in order to tell a story. Well, it seems that they have been set free. The art that they're creating is over the top amazing. As they worked today we left the classical music behind and moved on to Michael Jackson and other pop artists. They loved it. They danced and laughed while intensely creating the art that they are so passionate about.

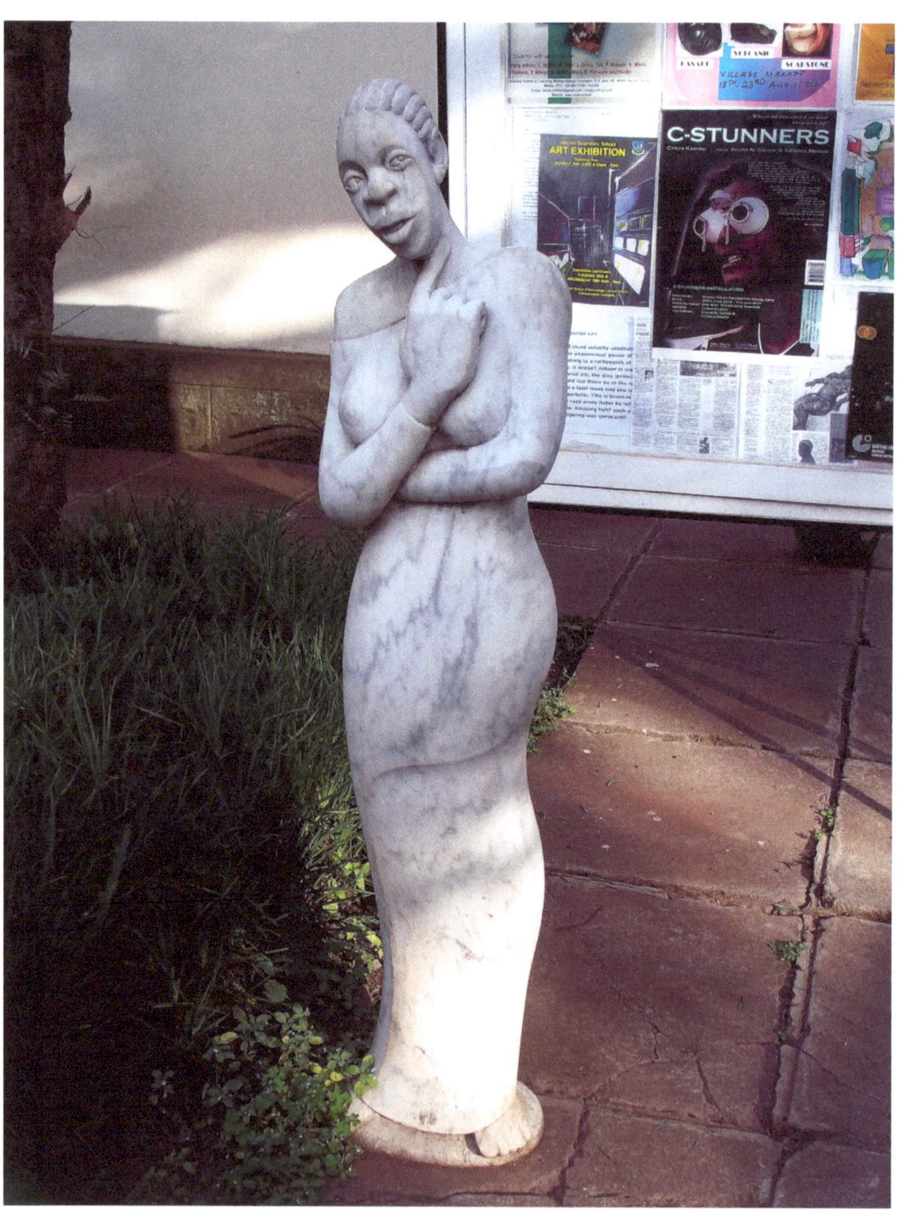

Kuona Trust

Surprisingly, my Form 2 class came early and wanted to start right away, so I set them up in another room. They are a very independent bunch. They are very connected to their work and seem content to repeat and repeat and repeat, which is really what helps an artist become more skilled; and then give them freedom and watch out.

Margaret's classes are robust and creative. The Form 3 class is using colors and forms and shapes and scenes that are just beautiful. She has been with this class for three years and watched them go from rowdy freshman to maturing juniors. Margaret handles their idiosyncrasies with such finesse and they respond to her tone and control of the class. The difference between Forms 3 and 4 is maturity. It is visible what a difference a year can make.

Her Form 1 class has a very different temperament and the drawing bug has really taken a bite out of them. More than any of the other classes thus far, they got it, they like it, they want it and they continue to flourish. Their portraits and the faces they draw– particularly their use of shading - are amazing.

After class we went to Kuona Trust for Cyrus Kabiru's exhibit called ***C-stunners*** which is an exhibit of eye glasses made into art. We each bought a pair of the art-glasses; they are so cool. We also met the head of the Kuona Trust, Danda Jaroljmek. She was engaged by the art of our students, the partnership of the trust with our program and by the possibility of coming to meet us (and others) in the US. She would like to find a way to engage the students of St. Al's regularly. It was just wonderful to be meeting members of the arts community in Nairobi. We also bought art from and visited with Fred Abuga, another great artist we met at Kuona Trust. All the people there are so gracious and engaging and well, just good people to know.

Tomorrow is our last day of class and then Friday is celebration day. In addition to our usual program, we'll be joined by the Thom Ogonga, head of school programs for the Kuona Trust and a freelance art correspondent who will be viewing the work of our students. They will be so excited.

Hope all is well, thanks for following us.

Charles and Margaret

THURSDAY, JULY 1, 2010
Last day of class, Frank Lloyd Wright and wow.

The last day of classes always ends up feeling a bit like a race. We make certificates, buy soda, ginger snaps and get things done in advance so we don't up end worrying about it on our celebration day. Franco had meetings come up at his day job, which had called him back from vacation. Yes, they took our fantastic Franco away. Well, Franco's stand-in was late.

We ran our errands and then stopped at – you guessed it – Nairobi Java to meet with our dear friend and inspiration, Ken Okoth. Before we knew it the clock said it was 3:20! The race back to the school brought us to its front door a mere seven

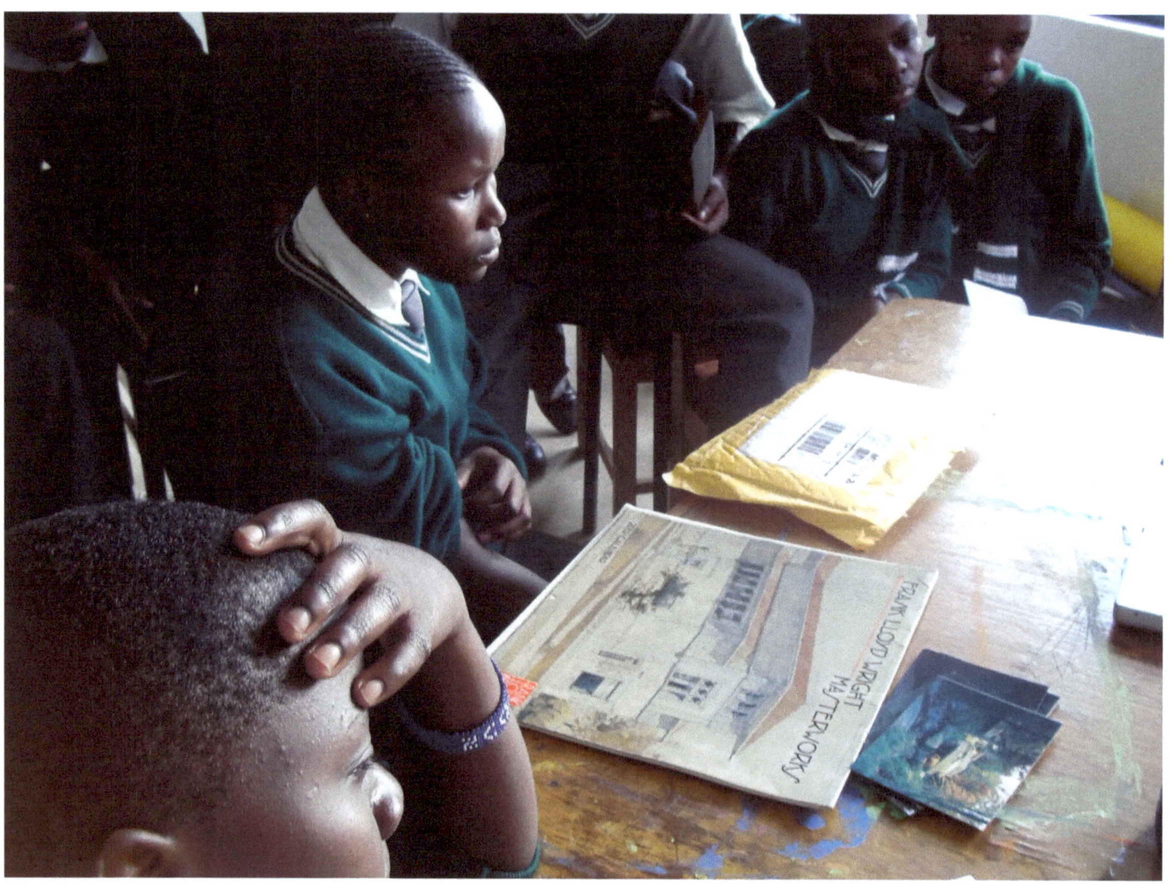

Students learn about Frank Lloyd Wright.

minutes before class was to begin. It was worth it. Ken, as I've shared with you, is one phenomenal human. He is so joyous and so affirming that we are doing the right things in Nairobi through our art program. Once we walked into the school, it felt like the sky cleared and the reason for our being there was right in front of us.....the Smart, Beautiful and Important Students of St. Al's.

Today was the day to deliver the presentation on Frank Lloyd Wright. We'd been waiting for the projector and computer with external modem all week. It took nearly half an hour to set up but to no avail. For some reason the presentation wouldn't stream over the principal's laptop and now the students were chomping at the bit because they really wanted to see it. Luckily, I had my six-year old Powerbook 12-inch computer, so we all gathered around its little screen watching and listening with rapt attention. I saw amazement on their faces. It was overwhelming to

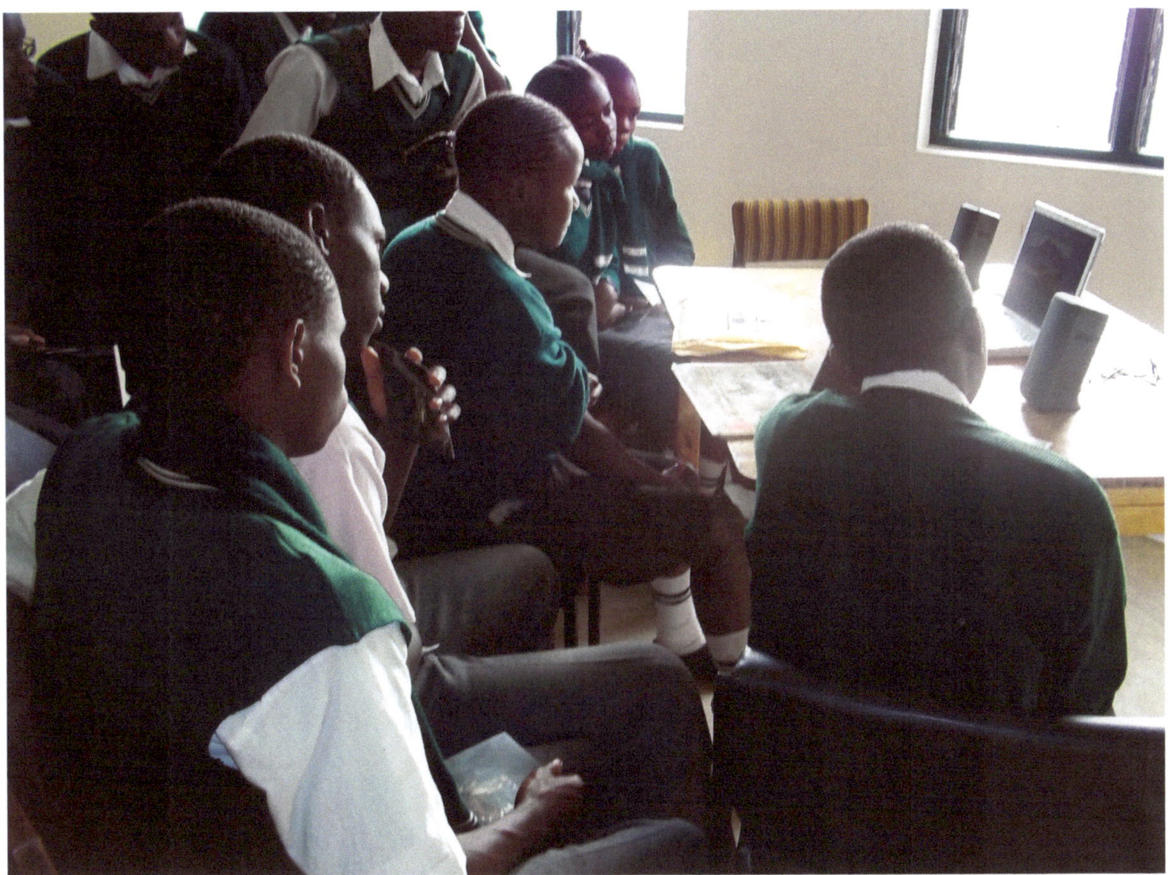

Watching a presentation on the work of Frank Lloyd Wright.

observe these students see the world unfold through Frank Lloyd Wright's unique vision. As a fan and admirer of FLW, watching the Form 4 class be overtaken by his creations, made me sit back and catch my breath. Watching them realize the house at Fallingwater, as someone in the class said, "lives on a waterfall" was unreal. When I gave them all post cards of the house they were overwhelmed, asking, "Is this for me? I can keep this?" It makes you realize how just a little goes very far. I also shared my pictures from my recent residency at Fallingwater with them and they loved them. They asked questions like, "why are you in the photo" and "how did you get there" like it was unattainable; I was powerfully reminded how this seems unattainable for not just my art students but for so many in the world. Thank you, Lynda Waggoner, Vice President of the Western Pennsylvania Conservancy and Director of Fallingwater and Justin Gunther, Curator of Fallingwater for sharing this privileged presentation and providing the post cards. The students loved it.

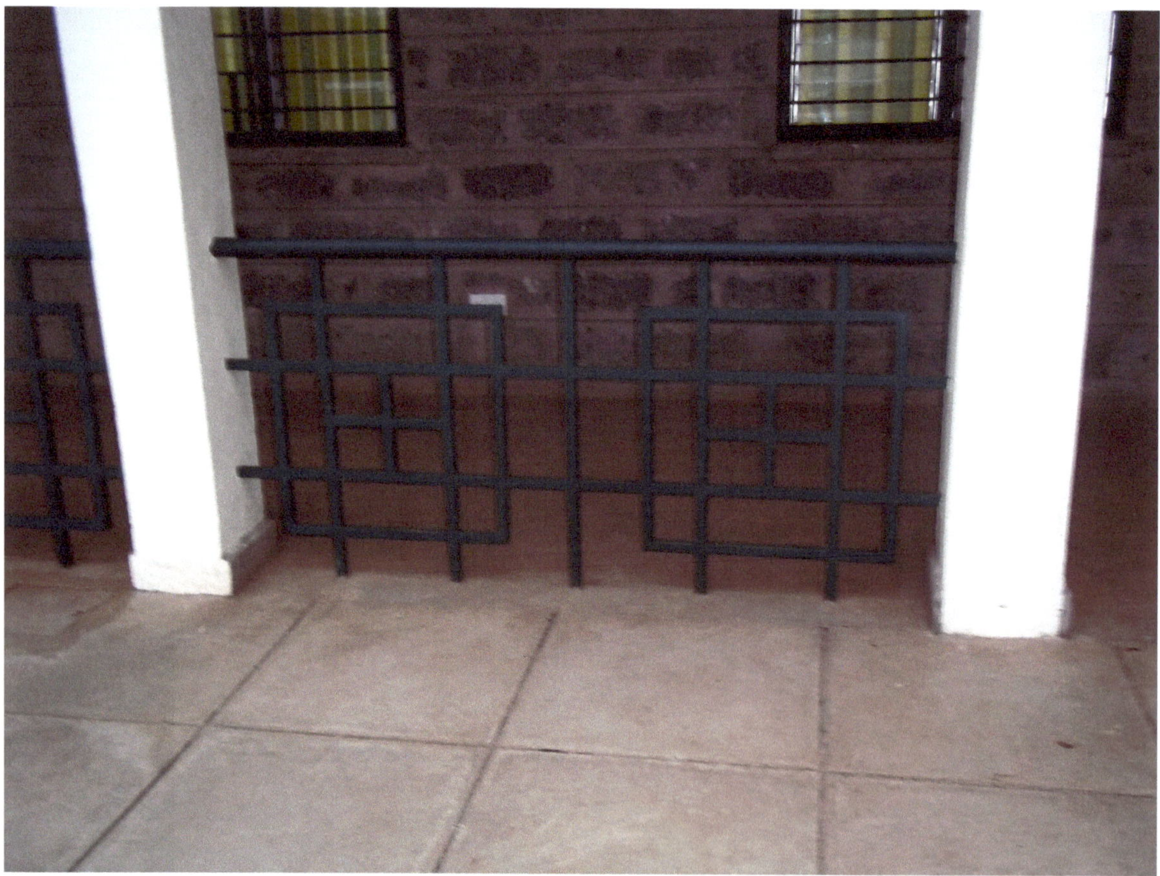

Could it be? A Frank Lloyd Wright-inspired design element at St. Al's?

As I was leaving the school, I was looking at the railings that run around the school and, if I did not know better, the new school looks like Frank Lloyd Wright had some influence in its design.

After the FLW presentation, the class dove into work on everything from watercolor to charcoal in their newly free style; some even did FLW-inspired work. Today, they were singing along to my – don't laugh -Glee soundtrack and nearly had to be thrown out fifteen minutes after class was officially over.

My Form 2 class usually starts at 5:15 but they wanted to start an hour early today. Being fiercely independent, they came in, took their supplies, asked for the key to their room, set up and asked when I might be by to provide instruction. Kelvin informed me that I needn't rush because they had lots of work to do. When I arrived they were focused on their painting or drawing and were ready to absorb all the new information I shared from artist bios today. This is my second year with this group and they are developing steadily. There is not one student that shines more brightly than the others, as in some of the other classes, but there is lots of talent.

Margaret's classes are producing in a way we didn't anticipate. Her Form 3 class - which she's been with from the start - still needs more focus and maturity, but they are diligent and some of their work is really stunning. The shapes, figures and colors that Saisi Wycliffe uses continue to amaze. He totally gets color and yet doesn't get it at all, and that combination results in some really beautiful art. He reminds me of Gauguin.

Margaret's Form 1 class demonstrates more potential then any of our other classes did during their first year. They are focused, quiet, and productive and damn good. They went from drawing to filling in their work with color today without direction. They listen to Margaret like she's delivering the state of the union or the sermon on the mount or something. Whatever she's saying, they recognize it as a message they need to hear. It is so heart warming and charming to see this group respond to her and to see the work they're producing.

As is now our routine, the end of each day of classes culminates in Margaret and me walking through all the classes together commenting on the artists' work; we have such pride in the work that they are doing. Margaret said something that has stuck with me, "At the end it always feels like they are just getting started." And she's right, it feels like that every year. However, I think we both take great comfort in the possibility that they'll build on the inspiration of these two weeks until we return next year.

Something occurred to me today. My Form 4 class started the program when they were in Form 2; this means that they won't get the full four years of the curriculum like all the other students will. Since there is a year between the end of secondary school and the start of higher education, I have committed to them that we will start the Graduate Institute for Art Immersion, which will serve as a bridge for them between high school and college. In 2011, the Graduate Institute will have the same curriculum that be delivered to Form 4, but in subsequent years the curriculum will be expanded beyond what's offered to Forms 1 – 4. I am sure that we can deliver it at St. Al's, but if not, Kuona Trust would love it if we did this type of work with them. We have options. This is exciting stuff.

I hope that you, dear readers, experience the absolute fulfillment that Margaret and I get out of this aspect of our lives. It is powerful, tangible and makes a difference. I never knew that we would be helping out Kenyans by providing them a venue to express themselves through art. We feel so lucky.

Be well.

Charles and Margaret

FRIDAY, JULY 2, 2010
Celebration Day. Our last day with the artists.

As always, this is a wonderful day, but it's also difficult. We got to the school early to have our closing meeting and debrief with Principal Beatrice and discussed the possibility of Kuona Trust coming monthly to provide an art "in session" for the students; we also talked about storing the art supplies and the idea of implementing The Graduate Institute. Beatrice is continually amazed at the work of the students and really demonstrates her excitement and support by giving us so much trust and latitude to make this all happen.

After our meeting, we each set up our rooms for celebration. Then Forms 3 and 4 arrive ready to celebrate, be rewarded and look at each other's art. To hear the

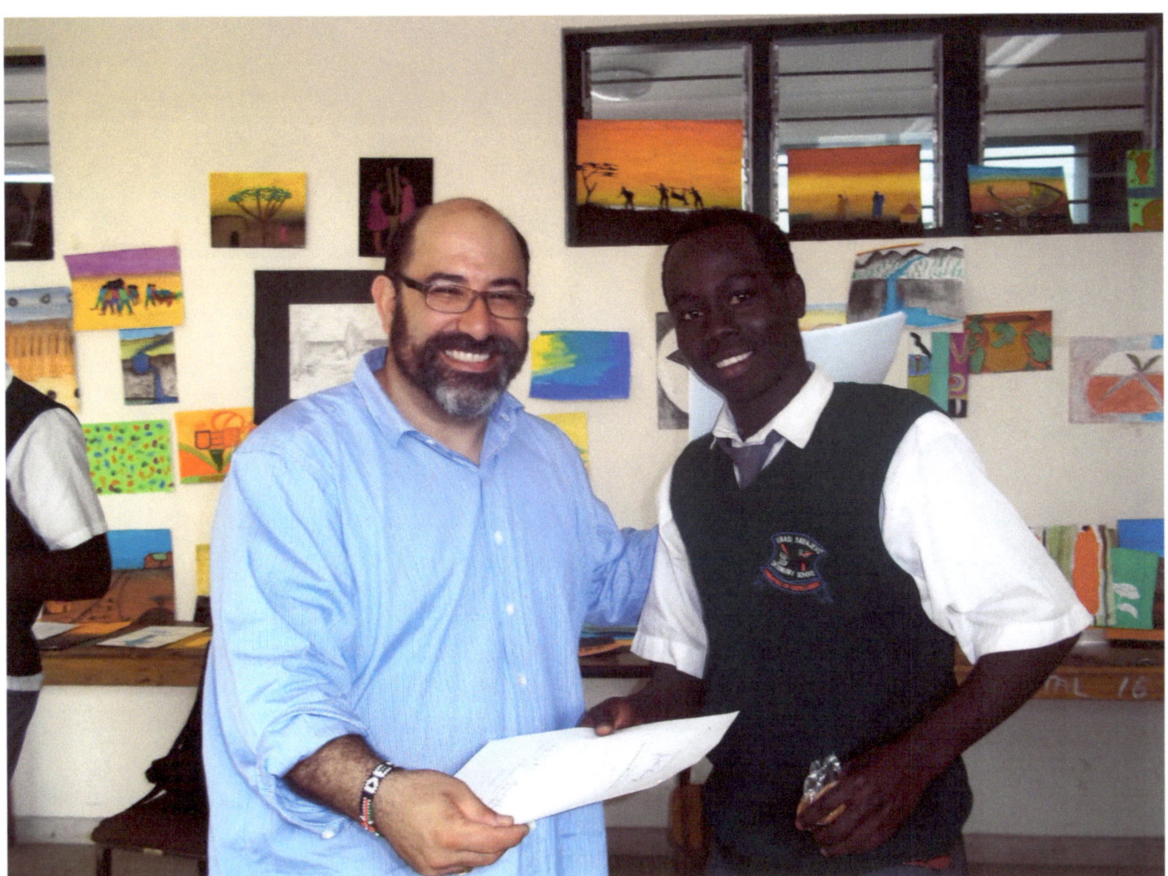

Passing out certificates on celebration day.

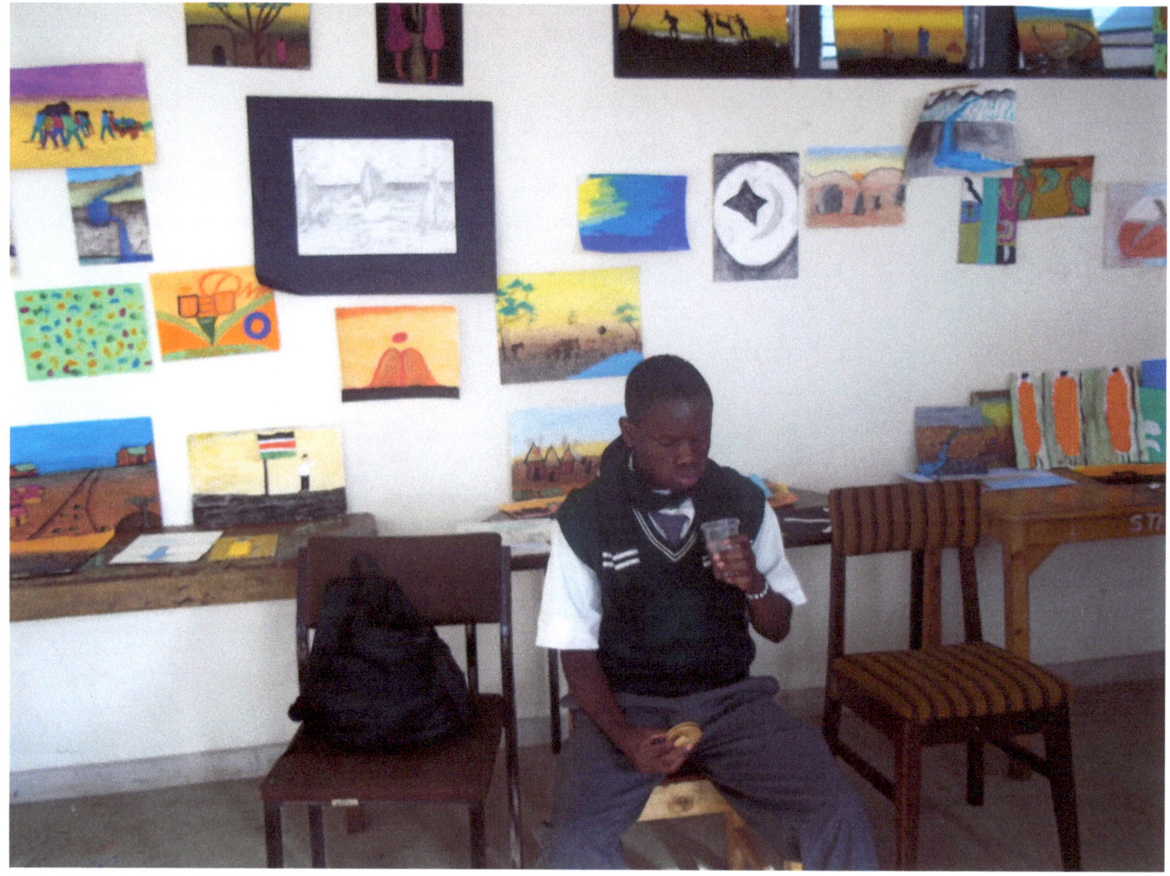

Ginger snaps and art go well together.

students discuss the art so maturely—its meaning, their emotional responses to it—was so pleasing to Margaret and me. They've become immersed, this is truly part of who they are now.

Today, Thom Ogonga of Kuona Trust was a guest in the class and it was so wonderful to see his reaction to, and interaction with, the students. He really loves working with student artists, something that he does on a regular basis in his role at the Kuona Trust. The students received their certificates with pride, had their soda, ginger snaps and cookies, milled around, danced to music, sang to me, loved on Margaret, said beautiful things to us and made us feel like we had been over paid for what we do. Really, we get so much from this.

True to form, my Form 2 class came early so they could prepare for the celebration; they hung their work and waited patiently. When their time came, we looked at their art, gave out certificates, had snacks and celebrated. It's really

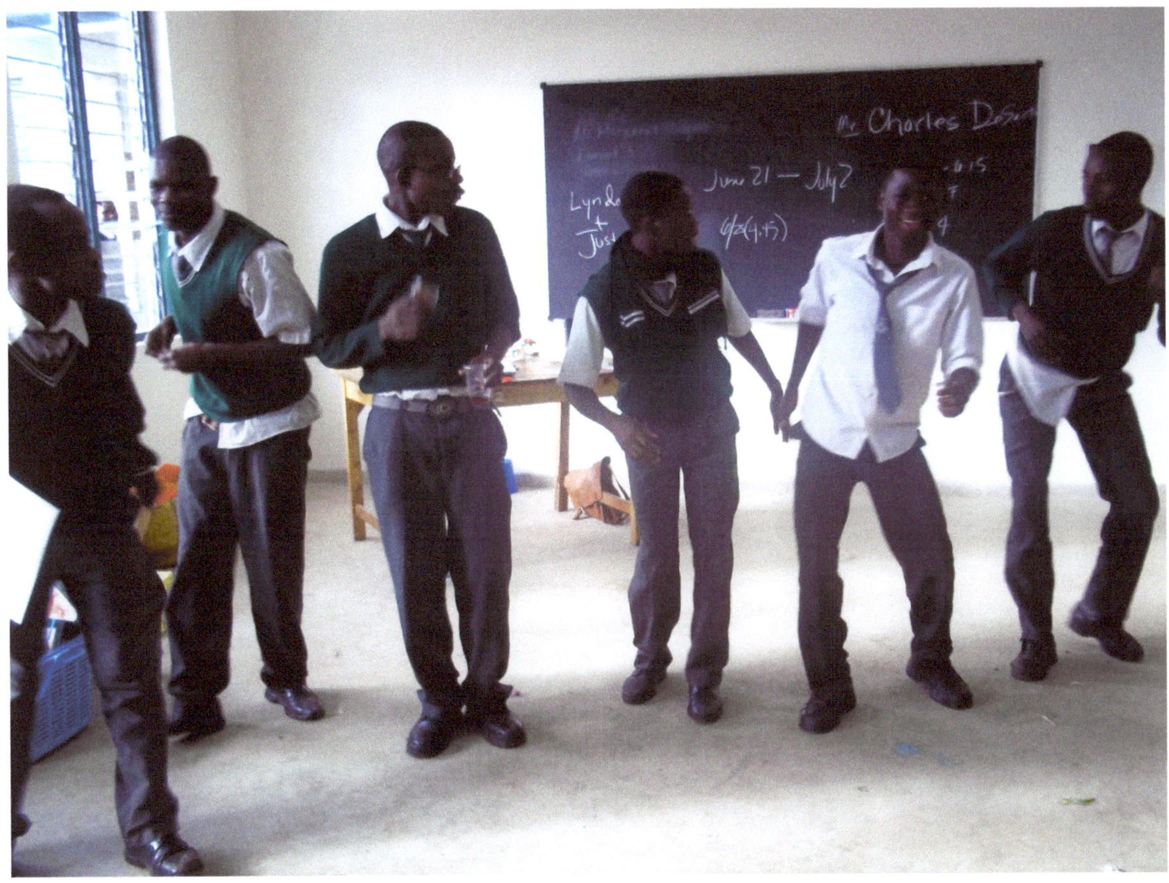

Students dance and celebrate on the final day of the Art in Kibera program.

exciting to think that they have two more years in which to develop and hone their skills. They are already well on their way to becoming powerful artists. They were happy and excited and said they couldn't wait to see me next year.

Margaret practically had to kick out the Form 3 class to make way for the Form 1 group to begin their celebration. As I've mentioned, this class seems like a higher caliber student at that age and they are truly ready to be the next big artists of St. Al's. Although my Form 4 class is really talented, I can't wait to see what this group will be producing in three more years.

Margaret's Form 3 class made her a video which I am sure she is watching as I write this; we each got lovely well wishes from our students, a few cards and lots of expressions of excitement for what they've accomplished and what is to come.

All in all, a day of absolute perfection followed by a celebratory dinner with Anne Wangari at the Norfork Hotel. It was an absolutely beautiful way to end our visit. Tomorrow, we'll have a day of fun before we leave late in the evening. We'll be taking the Georgetown graduate students to see the elephants at Sheldrick. This is an elephant rescue that everyone should see; it's so much fun. Then we will do whatever last minute running around we need to do before we depart Nairobi.

As I reflect on today, I see that Kenya continues to become not only more a part of our lives and reality, but a part of who we are. Thank you for being with us on this trip and indulging us by reading these blog entries. Knowing that so many of you share our interest and passion is enough to inspire us stateside as well as here in Africa. As I type this, Ghana is winning their match in the World Cup and I can hear cheering coming from the households across the valley. Just imagine the impact it would have on Africa if Ghana won the World Cup? Today I heard that, for the African people, it would have the same impact that Obama winning the presidency had on the Kenyan people.

Much Gratitude and look forward to seeing you soon,

Charles and Margaret

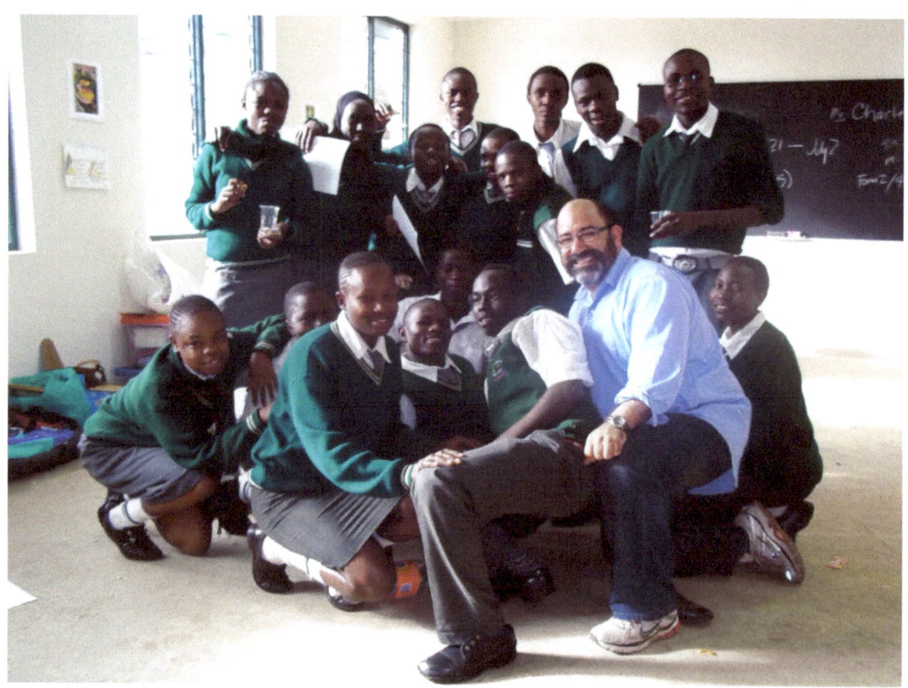

Graduating Form 4 students will be the first to have the opportunity to enroll in 2011 Graduate Institute.

WITH GRATITUDE

To Drs. Phil Boroughs, SJ and Kathleen Maas Wiegert, for inviting me to take part in the 2007 Kenya Immersion Trip. The experience changed my life beyond my wildest imaginings.

To Dr. Spiros Dimolitsas, for bringing me to the hilltop and allowing me to be part of a community that is so much more than a place to work; for believing in and empowering me to do not only the job you brought me to Georgetown University to do but so much more.

To Dr. Jack DeGioia, for creating an environment that not only encourages but requires global engagement; for embodying the Jesuit values of men and women for others within and well beyond the gates of Georgetown University.

To Clint Brooks, for your unbridled enthusiasm for this program; for the trust you placed in me as host to you and your two sons, Dillon and Timmy, during your own Kenya experience in March 2009; and for your always generous support.

To Rich and Teri Gendron, for your generous support and friendship.

To Dr. Beth Plunkett, whose unconditional love and friendship supports me in everything I do.

To Ben Quest, who always believes in me.

To Dr. Carole Sargent, your guidance and connections made this project a reality.

To Dr. Jim O'Donnell, for believing in my work in Kenya and for connecting the dots that made this book possible.

To Dr. Anna Lawton, my publisher at New Academia Publishing, for allowing this project to flow with such ease and believing in the Smart, Beautiful and Important students of St. Al's.

To the Office of Faculty and Staff Benefits at Georgetown University, for being the most amazing team of colleagues I could wish for; for allowing me to go to Kenya each year knowing without a doubt that you are fulfilling our mission of Choice, Access and Service, regardless of where I am in the world.

To Margaret Halpin, for being the yin to my yang since this program began in 2008; for believing, as ardently as I do, that art makes a big difference in people's lives.

To Anne Wangari Ndirangu, for bringing grace to my life; for allowing me to be part of your life, your family and your Kenya. I am truly honored.

To Rachel Bridges, for editing this book with such passion. Without you this project would have never been completed.

ABOUT THE AUTHOR

After living many years in San Francisco, Charles DeSantis moved to Washington, DC in 2006 after being recruited to serve as Associate Vice President and Chief Benefits Officer at Georgetown University. Charles travels frequently, from Africa to Italy, but ultimately enjoys the sanctuary of his little yellow carriage house in Georgetown that he shares with the lovely basset hound, Bella. There he can be found entertaining friends and neighbors, serving his famous vodka rigatoni, copious bottles of wine and fine chocolates.

www.ingramcontent.com/pod-product-compliance
Lightning Source LLC
LaVergne TN
LVHW071630100826
845154LV00007BA/125
* 9 7 8 0 9 8 2 8 0 6 1 1 1 *